Sirtfood Diet

Step-by-Step Guide to Cooking Healthy Dishes and Losing Weight Quickly With the Sirtfood Diet

Caled Reed

nature of this work, the Publisher is exempt from any responsibility of actions taken by the reader in conjunction with this work. The Publisher acknowledges that the reader acts of their own accord and releases the author and Publisher of any responsibility for the observance of tips, advice, counsel, strategies and techniques that may be offered in this volume.

Table of Contents

Introduction

Are you ready to lose some weight but do not know how? Perhaps you've tried losing weight on other diets in the past, but no matter how much you tried, you found that you either regained the weight or never lost it in the first place. Most diets that tend to trend are not very useful to most people—they simply are too restrictive, limiting, or ineffective due to how they work. Whether because they were too difficult to comply with or they are not meant to be long-term solutions to weight management, many of these options simply are no good for you. However, just because the latest crash diet that promised instant results did not pan out doesn't mean that you are stuck at whatever weight you are currently at. You can lose weight, and you can do so in a way that is healthy and without cutting out all of the foods that you may enjoy.

There are many diets to choose from, but one that is getting plenty of attention at the moment is the sirtfood diet. This diet focuses on sirtuins—proteins in foods that work to provide your body with a weight loss boost that will help you to achieve the success that you were looking for with yourself. This diet has been lauded by celebrities. Singer Adele recently claimed that she lost almost 100 lbs. on the sirtfood diet, using the green juice that we will be discussing, along with exercise. Through using sirtfood-rich foods in your diet and enjoying them regularly, you can unlock fat loss ad aid in preventing yourself from suffering from all sorts of diseases. You can make sure that you are as healthy as possible by making sure that your diet is as smooth as you can get it.

On the sirtfood diet, you will utilize sirtuins—those proteins that will help your body to regulate its metabolism. There are certain plant-based foods that are known to be loaded with sirtuins and, therefore, are believed to be the key to losing weight quickly. And, those foods that are rich in sirtuins are delicious as well—strawberries, dark chocolate, green tea, and even red wine are loaded with these higher levels of sirtuins that you can enjoy to help yourself feel good while eating healthy foods that will keep your energy levels boosted.

Though there are options that can help you lose weight without utilizing these powerful sirtuins, why not take advantage of a way that your body naturally works? Through consuming those sirtuin-rich foods, or "sirtfoods," you can begin to lose weight quickly and readily, especially when you exercise and restrict calories. As a result, you will be able to lose weight, and with the sirtfood diet, it has been found that people lose weight while still maintaining the same muscle mass they had before, meaning that they stay healthy and strong, regardless of the weight loss. Usually, during weight loss, there is a reduction in muscle mass that can be highly problematic to those who are trying to maintain their strength.

Now, you might be thinking that this sounds too good to be true—can you really lose the weight and still walk out with all of your muscle mass? Yes!! And, it is as simple as following this diet! Within this book, we will be going over the keys to unlocking this weight loss with ease, and all you have to do is figure out how to utilize the sirtfood diet and make it happen for you. Through making sure that the sirtfood diet is something that you can latch onto and then through providing yourself with the tools to do so, you can also achieve this weight loss. Remember, food is fuel, and we must eat certain foods if we want to survive. However, you should also enjoy it while you do so! There is no reason that the foods that you eat cannot be enjoyable, and for that reason, you will have this guide here to provide you with all sorts of foods that you can eat and prepare with ease to get the weight loss effects that you are looking for.

Within this book, you will be learning the ins and outs of the sirtfood diet, discovering everything that you will need to know about the diet itself and how it works. From there, you will discover what the most potent superfoods that you should enjoy are and why they matter. You will learn all about why you should always choose to consume certain foods over others and how they are so good for your body. We will also be addressing how to stick to the sirtfood diet, which has a very specific pattern that you are to follow to provide yourself with the right added effect. Finally, you will be provided several recipes that are meant to keep you as healthy as possible while still creating those effects that you are looking for.

At the end of the day, it is up to you whether you want to follow this diet or not. It is up to you whether you choose to follow along or if you want to move on to a different diet. Admittedly, this diet is quite strict, especially in the first week, but it does ease up, and you will find yourself able to enjoy several different meals and snacks throughout the day. All you have to do is reach out and start enjoying them!

Chapter 1: What is the Sirtfood Diet?

If you are still reading, then you are probably at least curious about what the sirtfood diet is and what you can expect from it. If you want to lose weight, you have probably already considered several different diet options, from the Mediterranean to the Paleo diet, but maybe none of them appeal to you. There is no shortage of diets out there that claim to be able to provide you with those instant weight loss results that you desire, but the truth is, nothing is instant, and nothing is free. If you want to lose weight yourself, then you will need to take the time to work for it, and you will have to choose a way that works for you.

If you had ever tried dieting before and failed, you probably know just how discouraging it can be to be in that position. However, if you want to learn how to succeed, you have to commit yourself. You can lose weight if you know what you are doing, and if you do so, you should also come to love the body that you are in as well. You deserve to be completely comfortable in the body that you have, and for that reason, you need a weight loss solution that works for you.

The sirtfood diet was initially designed in the United Kingdom by the celebrity nutritionists Aidan Goggins and Glen Matten. Together, they published their first recipe book in 2016 touting the power of activating the skinny gene. After all, some people seem to never gain weight regardless of what they eat, while others seem to pack on the pounds when they so much as look at a cookie. The difference, according to these nutritionists, may lie in the natural levels of sirtuins within the body. If some people have higher levels of sirtuins, then they are more likely to have an active metabolism.

As we go through this chapter, it is time to address the sirtfood diet in a bit more depth than we have been going through. We are going to address what the sirtfood diet is and why it matters. We will also address the benefits of the sirtfood diet, as well as who this diet is right for. Finally, we will wrap up by addressing some of the most common concerns with this diet and why some people may find that this is simply not right for them. Keep in mind that at the end of the day, before you start any diet, especially one as restrictive as the sirtfood diet at times, you should speak to your doctor and get their opinion as well. You want to make sure that your diet is something that is going to work for you, and the best way to get that is by having your doctor, who knows you and your body, approve.

What is the Sirtfood Diet?

Celebrated by people all over the internet, the sirtfood diet claims that through drinking green juice (more on this later!), eating sirtfoods, and exercising, weight can be lost rapidly, and even better, the weight can be kept off as well. It utilizes this idea of sirtuin-rich goods to kick-start the body's metabolism. By eating those sirtuin-rich foods, you will build up the level of sirtuins present in your body, and that will then allow you to burn more weight with ease.

This diet is relatively restrictive—you must change up what you are eating, and in some instances, you will be eating as little as 1000 calories per day for a period of time before easing up and starting to consume more. This is to get your body working and make sure that at the end of the day, you will be enjoying the added benefits of losing weight while still enjoying the foods that you get to consume. Many of the sirtuin-rich options are not only incredibly nutritious but also incredibly delicious as well. Foods such as blueberry pancakes, curried salmon, and the like are all allowed on this diet and will allow you to enjoy eating, even if the amount that you eat is different.

The sirtfood diet is, at its simplest, going to utilize calorie restriction while also boosting the number of sirtuins in the body. Through this two-pronged approach, and then implementing exercise as well, the end result is that you have the weight loss you need.

The Benefits of the Sirtfood Diet

This diet is filled with all sorts of benefits that will help you to achieve health and wellness. However, keep in mind that this diet is still being researched scientifically, but current evidence suggests that there are still benefits to the utilization of sirtuin activation and healthier foods. It is believed that there are many compelling benefits that make this diet a cut above the others and something that will provide you with plenty of health for yourself. Ultimately, when you work through this diet, you should find yourself getting benefits such as the following.

Losing weight

The most obvious benefit is the loss of weight over time. Whether you are actively exercising or you skip that step, this diet requires you to restrict your calories down to between 1000 and 1500 calories per day, depending upon the phase that you are in. When you consider basic math and the fact that the average person uses around 2000 calories per day, you see that this diet is going to cause a pretty extreme calorie deficit. By doing so, you will see that weight gets lost relatively quickly.

Weight loss is simple math—if you cut down your calories to well below what your metabolism is burning, you will naturally begin to lose weight. That weight, however, is normally a combination of both muscle and fat. As you lose weight and muscle, your metabolism also starts to slow down because there is less muscle to activate the metabolism in the first place. This means that over time, your metabolism drops with your weight, and eventually, you will get to a point where you have to cut even more calories or risk a plateau in your weight. Now, ideally, that plateau would occur at your healthy body weight, but that is not always the case. Sometimes, you will find yourself stagnant in your progress but still at an unhealthy weight, even with the caloric restrictions. This happens when your metabolism adjusts to the level by which you have cut your calories during all of that weight loss. Because usually, you will be losing muscle whether you want to or not, you will have to increasingly cut calories during your journey.

However, when you utilize the sirtfood diet, you will actually help prevent this. You do not usually lose much muscle mass while using this diet and that means that you do not have to deal with those implications. Because your muscle mass should stay relatively stagnant, or even grow in certain situations, you do not have to worry so much about your metabolism dropping as well.

Your appetite slows down

The first few days of this diet will likely be brutal. There is no way around it: Those first few days, you will dramatically restrict calories, and above all, you will also be cutting down the fiber content in your calories as well. That first phase is noted by the fact that you will be consuming juice (meaning that the fiber that you would normally have to bulk up your stomach will not be present) and a single meal per day. This can be tough when you first start your diet, but it is important to get the right effects. As a result, however, you will see that your body has to adjust to the caloric restrictions as well. You will have no choice but to adjust, and very quickly, you will discover that though you are eating less, you are not as hungry as you were before. You will be bulking up on healthy options that will keep you fuller for longer without requiring you to eat nearly the same amount.

You actually BUILD muscle

The sirtuins that you consume on this diet not only keep your muscle mass up, but studies have shown that sirtuins actually boost muscle mass as well. In a study done on aging mice, it was found that a sirtuin-rich diet actually allowed for the mice to grow more muscle and blood vessels, boosting energy by up to 80% at times. That increase was created simply by changing the diet. Yes, this is in mice and not people— but it is also incredibly promising. Mice are regularly used for studies on how things will impact people, and that implies that a similar effect should be noticeable for you as well. All you have to do is start switching up your diet and consuming more sirtuins.

Your blood sugar will stabilize

Another great benefit that you will see in most of these foods is the stabilization of blood sugar as well. This is due to the fact that sirtuin-rich foods tend to inhibit the release of insulin when you are in a state of fasting, which then allows for blood sugar to be stabilized. By using sirtuin-rich foods in your diet, you are able to keep your blood sugar from becoming too low or high, allowing for that management. Because insulin is responsible for breaking down the glucose to allow it to be used and because it is inhibited on this diet, your blood sugar stays right where it is supposed to for longer.

It is high in antioxidants

This diet is incredibly high in antioxidants. The ones provided to you in your sirtfoods that you will be consuming can actually create a great effect of treating the body and ensuring that you are able to avoid many common issues such as cancer or other chronic diseases. This is because antioxidants protect your body from free radicals, harmful waste byproducts that are created when your body functions. In particular, free radicals are formed when you break down food to digest it. As a result, you can wind up with all sorts of issues. Those antioxidants will actually prevent that damage, however, by helping to remove the free radicals that you have in your body.

Free radicals are commonly associated with ailments such as cancer, Parkinson's disease, arthritis, strokes, and many inflammatory conditions as well. However, when you consume the sirtfood diet, you are loading yourself up with those healthy antioxidants. By doing so, you provide yourself with recourse for your body to use to treat the problem entirely.

Additionally, the high prevalence of antioxidants may also be anti-aging. Because of the increase in muscle volume as well as the reduction in risk of many diseases, you can actually start to see that you stand a good chance of being able to help slow down the aging process to your body when you consume these foods. They are incredibly healthy for you—and all you will need to do is choose to consume them.

Is the Sirtfood Diet Right for You?

Of course, at this point, you are probably wondering whether this diet is going to be good for you in the first place. Is this diet right to help you? Do you even want to follow this diet? These are good questions to consider—and you will need to pay close attention to your own personal feelings. Remember, diets shouldn't leave you miserable or make you feel like you are in prison. You should have a diet that you are comfortable or willing to use if you want to actually lose the weight. After all, if you have a diet that you do not want to follow, you are significantly more likely to slip up the first time that you decide that you are uninterested in following it. What are you going to do if someone offers you a piece of cake and you've been miserably attempting to follow your diet? Chances are, you are going to find yourself miserable and not bothering to stick to it at all.

Are you someone who really has difficulties planning things out and sticking to them? Have you tried repeatedly to follow a diet plan, only to forego it as soon as things got tough? If so, this diet might not really be for you. You will need to be diligent in following through with this diet if you want to actually see the results that you want. You have to have the motivation and willpower to stick to things long enough for them to pay off, and when they do start to pay off, you will see that things get significantly better as well.

If you are someone who does not have any medical conditions that would make you a poor candidate for this diet, and if you are someone who is not going to have issues with sticking to the plan and having the willpower to turn down other foods, then this diet is a great one to try out. It can be incredibly beneficial, and all you need to do is find a way to get started.

Restrictions of the Diet

When you consume this diet, there are a few restrictions that you should consider and abide by. For example, when you are in the first phase of this diet, you generally are told to avoid red wine. Though red wine is commonly allowed during this diet, it is important to recognize that how alcohol breaks down is not going to help you during that time you are trying to kick-start your metabolism and getting it working for you.

You should also avoid eating processed foods during this diet. While this diet emphasizes healthy foods made at home, it is easy to stop and feel like you need to pick up a burger or something similar on your way home—and you should not be doing so. Because you want to make sure that your diet is healthy, and because you want to also make sure that you are restricting calories to get the weight loss you are looking for, you do not have any room in your diet for processed garbage that is going to keep you from getting the results that you are looking for.

The most important restriction, however, is the fact that you are restricting your calories significantly. During phase one, you can have just 1000 calories per day, and during the first three days of this, all you can consume is green juice and one meal per day. During the second phase of the diet, you can eat as much as you want, so long as you are mindful of the calories and keep them below 1500 per day.

Common Concerns

Of course, this diet is not an easy one to follow, and not everyone should attempt to follow this diet in the first place. When you follow this diet, you have to actually be healthy enough to sustain it. After all, being able to restrict your calories so significantly is a big deal. For the most part, most people should be healthy enough for this. However, there are certain people who may need to have some caution when they go through this diet to make sure that they do not overdo it.

For example, people with diabetes are typically not recommended to follow through with this diet. You will be juicing regularly, and that means that you will be removing all of the fiber that you need to keep your blood sugar levels more stabilized. If you are diabetic, then you can end up causing your body's blood sugar to spike and then plummet due to the lack of fiber to help regulate it. And, while it is true that the sirtfoods you choose out will help with regulating your blood sugar, you have to already have relatively stable blood sugar in the first place to be able to utilize that benefit.

Additionally, pregnant and breastfeeding mothers should not attempt to follow this diet. Due to the increased caloric requirement of mothers during these stages, it is important not to cut down on the calories when they matter the most. Your body will need you to provide the energy to either support the pregnancy or to provide you with enough to create breastmilk. Because of this, you will want to avoid this diet if those criteria qualify for you.

However, even if you do fall into the category of pregnant, breastfeeding, or diabetic, the truth is, you can actually still get plenty of use out of this book. You may not be able to restrict your calories, but you can still make it a point to follow the recipes. By modifying the way that you follow this diet, you can simply up your caloric intake while still enjoying these healthy foods that are going to keep you full and well-nourished. You will still be getting those healthy sirtuins, and that will still help you. You may just not see weight loss at the same speed.

What You Will Need

Now, you might be wondering what you are going to
need to keep on hand to follow this diet. And luckily,
all you really need, aside from the food, is a juicer. The
juicer is the most important tool that you can get—
because you are going to be juicing regularly, you
want to make sure that you have something high-
quality that will help you to process your ingredients
so that you will get the best possible benefit from
them. You want to make sure that you have something
that will process out the juice with ease and allow you
to get those benefits.

A good juicer will be somewhat pricy, but is a
necessary investment. A decent one is going to run at
least $100 if you buy it new. However, you may decide
that you want to invest even more to get the results
you want, and that is a perfectly viable option as well.
You just have to make sure that you have something
that is going to allow you to process your ingredients.
Ultimately, there are three main types of juicers:

1. **Centrifugal juicers:** These juicers are
    designed to quickly create juice for you to
    enjoy. They work with one large point where
    you can pour in your ingredients, and then they
    grate up the food that you put into them, using
    a sieve to extract juices that separate from the
    pulp as it spins. They are very good basic
    juicers that are quite simple to clean, but they
    are not the best out there. They are not always

as efficient as others, especially when working with greens.

2. **Masticating juicers:** These juicers work with a single gear that is used with an auger to grind and crush fruits and vegetables up. It is quite similar to the process of chewing food, hence the name. The juice is then separated out from the pulp and set aside. This type of juicer is the best for juicing greens and veggies, which is the primary use of this diet. However, they are also smaller and therefore require smaller pieces of food (which means more prep time!), and they may also take longer to make the juice.

3. **Triturating juicers:** These juicers are the most expensive options out there but are also top of the line. They work similarly to a masticating juicer with a slower motor and screws that interlock and crush up produce. When it comes to quality and getting the nutritional value you need, these are among the most effective of all. However, they are also quite slow.

Chapter 2: Does the Sirtfood Diet Work?

We've all see examples before. You know, where diets claim that they are the best and that they have the solution to some simple problem, or that they can help you lose weight quicker than any other. But, they never back up those claims. They never have anything to offer to assert these claims further, and as a result, you end up wondering why you even bothered trying them. However, keep in mind that this diet is not like the rest. When you are using the sirtfood diet, you are going to get real, tangible results rapidly due to the science behind how it works. And, this diet isn't about hiding the biomechanics behind how it works, either. You are encouraged to learn all about how this diet works for you, and the sooner that you start looking at it, the sooner you will succeed.

When it comes to managing your weight with this diet, you will be simply reducing the calories that you eat while boosting your activity levels. Additionally, you will be working on getting your body functioning better as well. You are looking for that added boost that will help you with that weight loss, and the sirtuins are responsible for it. Of course, we can state that as much as we want, but until you see the science, you may not be ready to believe this assertion.

Within this chapter, it is time to delve into how the sirtfood diet works and why it is so successful. The attempt from all ends to make sure that the diet is successful helps you to make sure that at the end of the day, you will be able to lose the weight without too much of a struggle. All you have to do is figure out what it is that you will need to do and then follow it. We will be going over sirtuins themselves first, and we will follow it up with the science behind caloric restriction and how it is so beneficial when you are trying to lose weight. Finally, we will address what happens to the body on this diet as well.

The Science of Sirtuins

Sirtuins are proteins within your cells that are there to regulate them. Typically, they are tasked with being able to maintain cellular homeostasis. This means that their jobs are to make sure that your cells stay exactly how they should be. They are meant to make sure that your body is consistent and that the consistency in your cells can be easily maintained. Because your body is designed to work within very specific parameters that are maintained during homeostasis, you need something to keep those parameters set. Just as homeostasis keeps your temperature just right to avoid allowing bacteria to run rampant in your body as well as your brain cooking if your body got too hot, sirtuins work within your body to make sure that you are kept within the right constant as well. The result is that you get a sort of cellular homeostasis.

The proteins within your body are like the workers—they keep your body functioning normally to make sure that you continue to live. Your body is full of several different functions and systems. You've got the nervous system, digestive system, respiratory system, and more. Each and every part of the body is meant to help with some degree of functionality, and ultimately, it is the proteins that help you to maintain this. It is the proteins in your body that will help to keep your organs running. Some proteins also have roles in keeping the other functions occurring while other proteins essentially manage them.

One way to better understand this is with the metaphor of your body being akin to a major corporation. Imagine that your whole body is analogous to one for a moment. Now, every particular organ or system is its own department. And, that means that sirtuins, in particular, serve their own personal role as their own department as well. They have one specific role: To release the fats in the body. When you let go of fats, you are able to start losing weight.

This works because all sirtuins work to remove acetyl groups from proteins. The acetyl groups within your body are there to alter and control how cells are responding to other cells. They work similarly to barcodes at a store—when they are scanned, it tells the computer exactly which product was scanned. Similarly, when acetyl groups are scanned, they tell other cells what to expect and how to engage. During acetylation, the process that sirtuins use, they reorganize the molecule to make sure that it is ready, and then, they activate the protein and send them off to work.

On the sirtfood diet, you fast and restrict calories. This tells your body to change how to respond to food. The sirtuins tell your body to respond differently. Instead of working to uptake the energy and store it as fat, your body is told to reject the fats, along with the cholesterol as well. As a result, your body burns the fats and cholesterol through oxidation. That allows the fat to be used up, burned, and then lost. This works to then allow you to lose the weight that you were trying to cut.

This works despite the restriction in calories. Most of the time, during calorie restriction, you run into the issue of your body trying to cling to any fat or sugar it can because it is unsure when it will get more. Because your body believes there is not enough fuel, it responds by cutting down how it burns the energy. As a result, you find your metabolism slowing down dramatically, and as it stops being as active, your body starts to pack on fat instead of burning it off. When you restrict calories, your body does not want to run out of energy. It works to prevent you from starving by slowing down how many calories you need. Of course, this is counterproductive compared to what your body wants and creates a situation in which weight loss becomes incredibly difficult. However, sirtuins can get past this.

If starving is seen as a threat to homeostasis, then the sirtuins should control it. However, because sirtuins want to keep things the same, they can then tell the body to continue functioning as normal. Through doing so, you end up seeing that the body continues to function at those higher levels. You see that the body is actually going to actively burn calories instead of clinging to them in the form of fat. The sirtuins will allow for the body to continue burning off that fat, and as a result, you continue to lose weight despite the severe degree of caloric restriction.

What Happens When I Restrict Calories?

Most diets work on a very simple premise: You cut down your calories to cause your body to burn the fat. After all, weight loss and gain are both simple equations: If you consume more calories than you burn, you gain weight, and likewise, if you burn more calories than you consume, you lose weight. It is that simple—so losing weight should be easy, right?

Unfortunately, it is not that simple, and there is significantly more to it than just that. When you restrict calories, you are actually conveying to your body that there is a problem that needs to be addressed, and the solution to that problem is actually counterintuitive. This is because your body loves homeostasis—it prefers to stay at the same state at all times without the fluctuations. Those fluctuations are believed to be problematic and should be avoided. As a result, your body chooses to cling to weight instead of losing it.

When you restrict calories, your body gets the message that there is no food available for it to consume. When you have a normal metabolism, it tells you when to eat and how much to eat to make sure that you constantly have the right level of energy to keep yourself stable. It's meant to help you stay on track and avoid running into a situation where you do not have enough blood sugar to function. Hunger is like the little gas light on your car—it turns on when you are starting to run low so you can correct it before you hit empty. When you get hungry, you need to eat to keep your calorie intake level so that you have enough energy to function.

However, when you cut those calories, you actually cut out the food that your body needs. As a result, you end up in a position where your body starts to shut down. It slows down the amount of energy that it burns through in an effort to maintain functionality longer. Yes, you have a backup of fat stores, but those are broken down relatively quickly, and they are broken down as soon as that deficit begins. This is how weight loss works—you cut your calories, so your body has no choice but to burn the fat to keep its stability. However, there are usually side effects to this, such as losing muscle with fat sometimes as well.

Calorie restriction is commonly treated by your body as a big threat, and for a good reason. However, if you were to work at it and implement those sirtfoods, you would see that your metabolism remains stable enough that you can continue to function relatively normally. As a result, you find yourself losing weight without seeing the speed of weight loss start to decline as well. This is perfect if you are trying to burn fat—it will keep your body burning off the fat at the same rate even those most other people would find themselves beginning to stagnate or simply not losing the weight at all. This is why the sirtfood diet is so incredibly powerful—it enables you to keep yourself functional and tap into your body to make it work the right way for you.

What Happens to the Body on the Sirtfood Diet?

When you choose to consume foods that are rich in sirtuins, you bring more sirtuins into your body. This, therefore, provides you with more access to them for breaking down and using them to create the fat-burning effects that you are looking for. You should see that the diet works better, the more sirtuins you consume. Even more beneficial, however, is the fact that the foods that you will see within this diet are actually incredibly healthy even aside from the fact that they are related to sirtuins. These foods are highly healthy and will allow you to keep your body running strongly.

The majority of the sirtuin-rich foods that you will be consuming are actually dubbed superfoods—they are full of nutrients beyond just the sirtuins that will have a phenomenal effect on the body and make sure that at the end of the day, you will have everything that you will need to thrive.

Chapter 3: A Guide to Sirtfoods

If you want to get started on the sirtfood diet, you will need to have all the right ingredients on hand so that you will be able to prepare foods that are right for you. Of course, this requires you to know what the best sirtfoods to have on hand are in the first place. Your diet requires you to eat mostly sirtuin-rich foods, and because of the fact that you are looking at meals that are going to be healthy and beneficial to you. You want to make sure that the foods on your list will matter and that everything that you put into your body is put there for a very important reason.

Especially due to the fact that your caloric allowance is slow on this diet, you want to make sure that you are getting the right foods to nourish yourself. You must make sure that the foods that you provide to yourself are going to provide you with plenty of good foods. Now, you might notice that this list is vegetarian; everything on this list in its own form comes from plants that you can enjoy. However, this is intentional—these foods are healthy and loaded with those sirtuins that you will need. Most sirtuins are found in these plant-based sources. What this means is that this diet is very compatible with both vegetarian and vegan diets as well if you want to follow them. Meat is not required for this diet.

But, before we get started on those recipes and meal planning, we will be looking at the ways that you can work on your own diet. We will be considering the foods that will give you the most sirtuin bang for your buck so you can prioritize them in your diet. Even if you find yourself choosing out foods that may not be included in the recipes here, at the very least, you will know that you have the option to enjoy these foods. You will be able to figure out what the best foods for you to eat on this diet are and how you can begin to implement them. This means that if you have recipes that you can make that are heavy in these foods, you should be able to enjoy them as well. By implementing all of these sirtuin-rich foods, you are also naturally consuming foods that are, for the most part, lower in sugar and lower in fat than most other recipes that you can make. This means that they are more likely to help you lose weight than other options for you and you can tap into that weight loss to make sure that you are losing the weight with ease. The more that you do this, the more likely you are to see those good benefits.

Arugula

Arugula is a very common vegetable. It is a leafy green that may also be written in some areas as "rocket," and it is quite similar to kale. It is used in much the same way that you would use spinach or other similar leafy veggies. It is one of the most potent superfoods that you can enjoy as well—it should be a part of your diet regularly. You can enjoy it with eggs, scrambled into it, or you can use it to help heal your body as well. In particular, arugula's big health benefit comes from the fact that it is loaded up with antioxidants that your body will use to heal. It can use these antioxidants to also keep your blood pressure and oxygen intake stable as well, and you can use it as a way to get some variety in your diet, especially if you are bored with kale. Or, you could use this food on its own. It is tender and mild, though some say slightly bitter and peppery. It can be a great addition to any diet and is incredibly healthy. Arugula is very deserving of its title as a superfood, and you will want to have this on hand at all times.

Bird's Eye Chili

Also regularly called the Thai chili, this is a chili pepper that comes from the *capsicum annuum* species. It is commonly found in both Ethiopia and Southeast Asia, and because of this, it is commonly found in many Asian cuisines as well. This pepper is quite spicy, rated on the Scoville scale between 50,000 and 100,000 SHU, making it quite potent. Jalapeno peppers, for example are up to 8,000 SHU while habaneros are usually rated at 100,000 to 350,000 SHU. This makes the bird's eye chili a potent addition to any dish, adding a great deal of heat. The heat that they possess comes from capsaicin, which may be spicy, but is also incredibly healthy. Capsaicin is actually found to be anti-inflammatory in nature and will provide you great benefits to eat it. However, if you do not enjoy spiciness, you can reduce the amount that you use, or you can also remove the seeds when you prepare the peppers for your recipes as well. The spiciness primarily resides in the seeds, so if you want to reduce the amount of spiciness that you consume, the best thing that you can do is cut them out entirely. You will also need to make sure that you protect yourself during the processing of these peppers. It is important for you to wear gloves to protect your hands, and you should also make sure that you do not touch your eyes or other sensitive areas of your body when you handle these peppers.

Blueberries

Blueberries are a delicious snack on their own. Who doesn't enjoy taking a handful of fresh blueberries, ripe and in season, and munching on them? They are sweet, but not overly so. And, they can be a great boost to your recipes that you may make, such as pancakes, muffins, or parfaits. Even in smoothies, these can be a fantastic way for you to enjoy the food that you are eating. All you have to do is keep them on hand! Of course, sometimes, they may not be in season, and in those situations, frozen berries work just as well.

Blueberries owe their superfood and sirtfood claim to fame to the fact that they are loaded with minerals that will help you to stay healthy. Sirtuins aside, they are also full of vitamin K, potassium, vitamin c, and all sorts of antioxidants that will help you to stay healthy. All you have to do is enjoy them! When you take the time to enjoy this diet, you will find yourself getting all sorts of benefits. These will be used regularly in many of the dessert dishes that you have, and if you want to snack on them, you should! You will get great benefits!

Buckwheat

Buckwheat is a type of seed that is typically called pseudocereal, and it will be a primary substitute for most grains in your diet. You will be able to enjoy buckwheat processed into groats, noodles, flour, and more. It can be used much like rice, or it can serve as the flour base for baked goods. And, because it is a seed and not a grain, it is actually much healthier for you. It is also gluten-free and will provide you with a great, healthy source of carbs as well. In addition to the carbs, it is also high in protein and is low to medium on the glycemic index. This refers to how quickly your blood sugar level is raised in response.

Buckwheat is healthy thanks to the high fiber content, as well as protein. And along with that, it is high in minerals that your body can use to thrive. In addition, it is a fantastic source of antioxidants and sirtuins that you can enjoy as well. As you follow this diet, you will be able to get all sorts of health benefits that you can enjoy. In fact, you will have more antioxidant boosts in this ingredient than you would see in most other common cereal grains. In particular, you will get rutin and quercetin out of this particular dish. Rutin is the main antioxidant that is present in buckwheat and will lower cancer risk while also improving inflammation. Quercetin is an important antioxidant that has been found to be incredibly healthy and beneficial as well.

Capers

Capers are high in sirtuins as well. These are the small, unripened flower buds that come from the caper bush. Typically cultivated in the Mediterranean region along with Asia and Australia, this plant is commonly associated with providing a huge burst of flavor while also adding tanginess and texture to any dish. It is commonly found in pasta, sauces, and in fish recipes. This particular ingredient, despite being small and somewhat nondescript, is actually quite delicious. It is dried in the sun, then pickled to get the flavor familiar with it.

Capers are known to be low in calories, carbs, and fat, making them a great option for flavor. And, because they are high in minerals, you can usually get some great benefits from enjoying them. However, be mindful—they are high in salt content. If you do not know where you need to go for them in the store, try checking out the pickle area. You should find yourself getting those great benefits from enjoying them if you pick them up.

Coffee

For most adults, coffee is a staple in their diet. Who doesn't enjoy that boost of energy thanks to the caffeine? For many people on many diets that require them to cut out coffee, they find themselves dragging. However, on this diet, you are recommended and even encouraged to enjoy coffee on a regular basis. Not only will it not add to your caloric consumption for the day when drank black, but it is also loaded with natural energy as well as antioxidants. The introduction of coffee to your diet will help you immensely.

Coffee is loaded with sirtuins as well and gives your body a boost to its metabolism as well. This allows your body to get that effect that you are looking for, and before you know it, you will be losing weight. Coffee is regularly favored by those seeking to lose weight just thanks to how it works—but be mindful that adding sugar or milk will cause it to lose out on most of these benefits. Coffee should be enjoyed black if at all possible.

Dark Chocolate

Of course, you are also going to want something sweet in your diet every now and then as well. Dark chocolate is the perfect option if you want that sweet baked good without having to worry so much about the foods that you are enjoying. Do you want a delicious mousse? You can get those if you use dark chocolate and tofu. What about a chocolatey coffee drink? Dark chocolate can provide that to you as well. Dark chocolate is a fantastic source of sirtuins that will help you to stay healthy, and it will also be great for you for other reasons as well. Science shows that dark chocolate is one of the best sources of antioxidants in the world, meaning that every time you enjoy that little sweet treat, you are feeding yourself a phenomenal superfood that is going to serve to benefit you immensely.

This is thanks to the nutritional content found within high-quality dark chocolate that is known to have a high cocoa content. When you get dark chocolate that is 70-85% cocoa, you are providing yourself some fantastic benefits in the form of:

- 11 grams of fiber
- 58% of the RDI for magnesium
- 67% of the RDI for iron
- 89% of the RDI for copper
- 98% of the RDI for manganese
- Plenty of potassium, phosphorus, zinc, and selenium

Of course, those benefits come along with 100 grams (3.5 oz.) of chocolate, and you will probably not be eating this much often. However, this is a huge nutritional powerhouse when you compare per calorie with the nutrition within them. Beyond those benefits, the high level of polyphenols, flavanols, and catechins make your dark chocolate highly beneficial. All you have to do is enjoy it in moderation.

Extra Virgin Olive Oil

When you cook, you will need some sort of fat. This is simply due to the fact that you will need something to prevent your food from burning, and you simply need fat as a part of your diet. Your brain, in particular, is highly dependent upon fat, and if you are not providing it for yourself, you will be unhealthy. However, those fats have to come from healthy sources. One such source is through the use of extra virgin olive oil. EVOO is one of the world's healthiest fats that you can consume, and it has so many different benefits. In fact, in many parts of the world where people use olive oil almost exclusively, people live longer and are healthier in general. This is one of the biggest things pushed during the Mediterranean diet—cook with olive oil.

In particular, you need extra virgin olive oil to get the true benefits that you are looking for. These are created through the use of extracting oils from olives without relying on heat or chemicals. It is purer and allows for most of the health benefits to be maintained to make sure that you are getting a healthy diet. EVOO is loaded with all sorts of good antioxidants and healthy fats that your body will require to stay healthy. Thanks to the more than 30 compounds full of antioxidants. This heart-healthy fat is loaded with benefits and will help you to stay well, all while also providing you with a delicious flavor.

Kale

Kale is one of the most nutrient-rich foods that you can enjoy in your diet. If you want to be able to enjoy these foods, you will be able to do so just due to the fact that it is so healthy. Kale is loaded up with all sorts of sirtuins and antioxidants that will help you to keep your health exactly as you need it. This will be a heavy part of your diet, as well. You can expect to consume it daily, as it does have a role in your juice that you consume each day. However, it is worth it— the benefits that you get are immense.

Kale can come in green or purple or may be curly or smooth. However, either way, you are getting those great benefits. One cup of raw kale is known to contain the following:

- Calcium: 9% of the daily value
- Copper: 10% of the daily value
- Magnesium: 6% of the daily value
- Manganese: 26% of the daily value
- Potassium: 9% of the daily value
- Vitamin A: 206% of the daily value (from beta-carotene)
- Vitamin B6: 9% of the daily value
- Vitamin C: 134% of the daily value
- Vitamin K: 684% of the daily value

With that nutritional load, you are only consuming 33 calories as well as plenty of antioxidants, meaning that when you consider the nutritional value to calorie ratio, you can't beat it. This is one of the best ways to get those added boosts without having to do much to your diet. You can get great results just by virtue of knowing how to adjust what you are eating and how you are consuming it. Replacing many of your greens in your diet with kale will be doing you a massive favor nutritionally.

Lovage

Lovage is an herbal supplement that is most known around the Mediterranean region of the planet. It is in the same family as plants that you are probably more familiar with, such as carrots, dill, and parsley, and the leaves will be quite reminiscent of cilantro. Though it has a strong smell to it, it is a pleasant, warm, and aromatic flavor. This plant is not commonly used in food but is recognized for its medicinal content, and because of that, along with its potency with sirtfoods, makes it highly popular in all sorts of contexts within this diet.

This herb, however, is recommended to be avoided if you are pregnant or intending to become pregnant as it may lead to miscarriage. If you believe that you are pregnant or you intend to become pregnant, you may want to skip this ingredient in any of the recipes that you do.

Medjool Dates

Another ingredient that you will see featured heavily is the Medjool date. This food will provide you with a ton of sirtuins while also providing so many different benefits with it. These are naturally quite sweet and will help you to avoid adding sugar to the foods that you are enjoying. You will see these used in brownie recipes and more, providing you with that sirtuin benefit while also providing you with everything that you are going to need to stay healthy.

These fruits are loaded up with all sorts of benefits and are delicious. In baking, they provide a great deal of sweetening while also cutting the calories and providing fiber as well. They are also great in salads and will be loaded up with potassium. They are actually 50% denser in potassium than even bananas. They are great, especially with the fiber included as well. If you want to enjoy them, in just 3.5 ounces of dates, you get the following:

- **Calories:** 277
- **Carbs:** 75 grams
- **Fiber:** 7 grams
- **Protein:** 2 grams
- **Potassium:** 20% of the recommended daily allowance
- **Magnesium**: 14% of the recommended daily allowance
- **Copper:** 18% of the recommended daily allowance

- **Manganese:** 15% of the recommended daily allowance
- **Iron:** 5% of the recommended daily allowance
- **Vitamin B6:** 12% of the recommended daily allowance

Matcha

Another primary part of the sirtfood diet is the use of matcha tea. This tea is great for keeping your health in order while also providing you with ways that you can improve your health. When you enjoy matcha, you are getting green tea that comes from covering the tea plants for the last month prior to harvest. As a result of depriving the leaves of direct sunlight, the production of chlorophyll in the plants grows, and there is a significant boost in the content of amino acids. This gives matcha its characteristic green color.

Additionally, because the creation of matcha also involves the use of the entire leaf, you actually get more caffeine and more antioxidants. This is why matcha is so popular on this diet- you get the boost of caffeine that will allow you to get that thriving functionality while also getting the benefits of protecting the liver, the heart, and aiding in weight loss.

Matcha's high antioxidant levels allow it to be particularly potent in providing you the benefits. This is why the leaves are powdered down to make tea— you get all of the nutrients from the leaf rather than just the result of steeping the leaf in water. It is believed that matcha actually contains up to 137 times more catechins than other green teas, and in studies that provided matcha to mice, it was shown that damage caused by free radicals was actually reduced. This means that by enjoying matcha, you are not only providing yourself with sirtuins, you are also providing yourself with benefits that will help you to protect your cells from free radicals as well.

Onions

Onions are a fundamental part of just about any cuisine, thanks to the intense flavor they impart. Onions are a great way to get that warm, strong flavor into your dishes without needing salt to add it. And, they are also incredibly rich in sirtuins as well. The very same vitamins and minerals that are responsible for the smell that onions have actually made them incredibly healthy as well. And, if you enjoy your onions with tomato and oil as well, you get the synergistic effect to create a rich powerhouse of all sorts of healthy vitamins, minerals, and fats that will help you to thrive. You will notice this regularly throughout many of the recipes provided to you—they are full of onion, tomato, and olive oil together.

Parsley

Though most people would not take a look at parsley and think that there is anything of real value in it, it is actually loaded with all sorts of anti-inflammatory and antioxidant value. In particular, parsley is an incredibly rich source of sirtuins and will provide you with all sorts of great benefits. Though commonly used as a garnish, you can get great benefits if you make it the star of some of the dishes that you consume. In fact, you will be featuring parsley heavily during your time following this diet. It is one of the primary ingredients in the classic green juice that you will be consuming several times. So, pack up on the parsley or learn to grow it yourself; you are going to need it to thrive and to get the best bang for your buck on this dietary journey. But, before you know it, you will be quite accustomed to the benefits that you will get. This particular ingredient is full of versatility and purpose that will be worth every bite that you take.

Red Chicory

When you want to fill yourself up quickly, you can enjoy some red chicory. Red chicory is loaded up with fiber, allowing for your guts to get that added prebiotic benefit. The fiber feeds the bacteria in your body and allows you to enjoy the benefits of having a healthy digestive system. And, you will be able to enjoy this food in other recipes as well. It can be enjoyed just like celery, or you could also choose to turn the roots and leaves into tea. Either way, you get some great benefits that will help your body thanks to the sirtuin content within it. At the end of the day, the sooner that you get those added benefits, the sooner

that you find yourself thriving. Red chicory can be added
To your dishes or used as a traditional medicinal treatment as well. In this diet, you will commonly enjoy it in your dishes.

Red Wine

Though alcohol is generally not a part of any healthy diet, certain diets recommend the added benefit of enjoying some red wine with your meals. In particular, the Mediterranean diet is famous for this, recognizing that red wine in moderation has enough benefits that it should be included. On the sirtfood diet, you also get the added benefit of getting to enjoy red wine thanks to the fact that it is actually loaded with benefits. In particular, it contains sirtuin-activating nutrients known as resveratrol and piceatannol. This means that adding a glass or two of red wine with a meal actually helps you to keep your body functioning and improves the ability of the sirtuins to actually be beneficial to your health as well. Beyond that, however, there are many studies that have shown that red wine is actually quite nutritious and that you can enjoy it in moderation. It has been found that small amounts of alcohol actually reduce the risk of death from cardiovascular disease and that people who drink moderate amounts of wine regularly actually see a 30% reduction of risk in heart disease. In moderation, meaning one or two glasses per day, you actually reduce the risk of health issues.

However, you must also be careful on this diet. You will need to make sure that you count your calories carefully because wine is naturally high in calories. This means that when you are so limited in terms of what you can consume, you will need to be mindful and count carefully if you really want to lose the weight on this diet.

Soy

One of the best sources of protein that you can enjoy on this diet comes from soy. Though some people dislike the inclusion of soy due to the phytoestrogen, which mimics the impacts of estrogen in the body, it is quite healthy for you. Soy is loaded with all sorts of vitamins and minerals, as well as the omega-3 and omega-6 fatty acids in the right ratios, ensuring that you are getting fat and protein while following this diet.

In particular, this diet will primarily feature tofu as a great vegetarian protein source. Of course, there will be other dishes as well that will include meats such as chicken and fish, but when given a choice, it is recommended that you take the tofu option if you want the best sirtfood options for yourself.

Strawberries

Blueberries are not the only berry that you will want to emphasize on this diet. Strawberries are also going to be a major star of the show in this diet, providing you with all sorts of great benefits. When you enjoy strawberries, you are filling up on nutrient-rich options that will be loaded in the vitamins and minerals that you will need to stay healthy, along with the sirtuins that you need for your weight loss. Like blueberries, strawberries are the perfect addition to your diet if you are looking for smoothies, yogurts, or even salads. They will provide you with those added benefits that you need and will taste good as you go.

Along with sirtuins, strawberries owe their health status to the fact that they are loaded with antioxidants while also being loaded with manganese and potassium. In addition, they are also free of sodium, fat, and cholesterol, as well as being low-calorie. The fiber levels also help to make sure that your blood sugar is kept consistent, and you are left feeling full. Give them a shot and enjoy your diet.

Turmeric

A common spice that is used heavily on this diet is turmeric. This particular spice is highly popular thanks to the fact that it is loaded up with curcumin—an antioxidant that is incredibly healthy for you, as well as anti-inflammatory. On this diet, you will be primarily focusing on this spice in many dishes, providing explosive flavor and fragrance to your meals. Thanks to the health benefits of this dish, you will regularly see people go for curried dishes on this diet to get the best bang for their buck. In particular,

the best benefits come from the fact that it can help
the body to regulate itself.

However, if you are using turmeric regularly, you
must make sure that you are also taking into
consideration the fact that it does stain. If you are
using turmeric in your diet, you will also want to make
sure that you are considerate of what materials you
use. Stick to glass and stainless steel if you are using
turmeric, or you may find that your dishes stain.

Walnuts

Finally, the last major sirtfood that you will consider
in your diet is walnut. This is a great source of fat for
you, loaded up with omega-3 fatty acids that are not
only good for your body, but are also great at keeping
you fuller for longer. They are incredibly beneficial
thanks to their high antioxidant content, elevating
them into superfood status, and as a result, you want
to consider the fact that the addition of walnuts can be
fantastic for you if you want to be able to provide
yourself with those benefits that you are looking for.

However, remember that walnuts, as healthy as they
are, must be used in moderation. This is because
walnuts are actually incredibly high in fat. The fat that
they have in them also means that they are incredibly
high in calories as well. This means that you need to
use them carefully on this diet or you can end up
unintentionally going over your caloric limits on this
diet.

Chapter 4: Sticking to the Sirtfood Diet

So, after taking a look at the foods available to you and starting to understand a bit more about this diet, are you ready to get started? Do you want to start reaping the benefits of this diet by enjoying them regularly? If so, then you are in the right spot. At this point, it is time to start going over the ins and outs of the sirtfood diet so that you can be certain that you understand what you will be committing yourself to. By following this diet, you should be able to provide yourself with all sorts of important benefits. You will be committing yourself to be willing to follow this diet for, at the bare minimum, two weeks to begin getting those benefits that you are looking for, and that means that you should have a good idea of what you will need to do.

Remember that this diet is not meant to be permanent, while the various foods that are recommended ought to continue to be present in your diet at higher levels than normal just due to the fact that they are going to provide you with all sorts of health benefits. When you are able to get through the diet, you will be committing to losing weight. But, you will also be committing to a healthier lifestyle as well. The foods that you enjoy on this diet are healthy for you and are still incredibly tasty as well. Yes, you might have a bit of an adjustment period if you are unaccustomed to consuming foods that are primarily based upon plants or that will use dark leafy greens. Some of these flavors are admittedly acquired tastes, but the diet can still be plenty enjoyable to you if you know how to go through it.

Before we dive into the foods that you can make on this diet, let's first consider the various aspects of it. Now, at this point, we've mentioned that the sirtfood diet involves two key phases that you must follow. However, there is more to it than just that—it is time to dive into how the diet works and why you have to follow it in the way that you do. You want to make sure that you follow each phase to a T if you want to be able to provide yourself with the touted benefits that you can get on this diet. However, doing so is not difficult—you just have to take the time and make it a point to figure out what it is that you will consume and why you will consume what you do. If you follow this, you should begin to see the benefits, and the weight will melt off.

Keep in mind that during this whole process, it is still strongly recommended that you stick to the exercise routine that you were doing before. Yes, you are cutting down the calories that you are consuming, but you still want to exercise if you want to get that benefit of cutting down the weight as well. It might be difficult in those first few days, but remember, this is temporary, and this will pass. If you want to get the results, you will have to put in the effort, and this book is here to help you to do just that.

As you read through this chapter, we are going to first emphasize the importance of the green juice that is used on this diet to provide you with the bulk of your diet in the early days. From there, we will be discussing the phases that go into this diet as well, going over what you can expect and why in both phases. We will go over what you should expect to do after completing the two-week cycle, and finally, we will wrap this chapter up with the tips and tricks that you should consider if you want to stick to diets in general. These tips are going to be relevant regardless of which diet you are on, and they will help you immensely on your journey of weight loss. Remember that at the end of the day, you control yourself. At the end of the day, you have the power to dictate how your diet is going to go and what your results are going to look like. If you can do so, you will find yourself thriving. Are you ready to start understanding everything that you will need to know on this diet? If so, then let's dive right in!

Sirtfood Green Juice

When you get through the sirtfood diet, one thing that you must do is consume green juice on a daily basis. You are not consuming just any green juice either—it is a very specific green juice that is designed to give your metabolism a burst of energy, kicking it into gear while also giving you plenty of nourishment to help yourself stick to your diet. Some people do not like green juice very much, but it is an important aspect of this diet when it comes to ensuring that you are consistent with your results. If you want to get the best benefits, you will need to have quality ingredients that will help you to thrive.

The green juice that you drink will be loaded with kale, arugula, parsley, lovage, celery, apple, lemon, and matcha, and together, you get a drink that is potent. You will be enjoying it several times a day in the earliest parts of your diet, but when you do so, you will start finding all sorts of benefits as well. At the end of the day, one of the best things that you can do for yourself will be to learn to love this recipe. However, if you are going to be consuming this drink in the evenings, it is important for you to remember that you should cut out the matcha. The matcha levels within the drink contain the same amount of caffeine as you can expect to find in a cup of coffee, so you will need to be mindful of how much caffeine you are consuming at any point in time, especially if you do not want to be kept up all night from a glass of matcha-loaded green juice.

You will notice that on every day of this diet, you are recommended to drink between one and three glasses of green juice per day, depending upon the phase that you are in. When you follow the recommendations, you will be bulking up most of the day on just green juice in the beginning, but even when you are done with following the phases of this diet, you should still include a daily glass of green juice in your routine.

Phase One

The first phase is undoubtedly the hardest part of it. When you are in phase one of your diet, you will have to consider the fact that you are looking to trigger the right state of your metabolism. You are trying to trigger your body to start using the sirtuins to their best benefit, which means that you have to deprive your body of calories while still providing plenty of sirtuins so that your body focuses on only burning fat without slowing down the immune system. After all, any diet that involves weight loss is going to be dependent upon caloric deprivation somewhere along the way.

This first phase is difficult because of the restrictiveness of it, however. The sheer restrictions are enough to make most people shy away from committing just due to the fact that you are cutting down your calories so much. Keep in mind that before you commit to anything, you should talk to your doctor to determine if cutting down your calories so much is actually going to be good for you in the first place. If you want to get that caloric cut that you are looking for, you need to drop down to 1000 calories per day. This is not something that is possible for everyone, however, so you will need to make sure that your doctor will approve of before you get started.

During phase one, there are two different parts that you will go through. The first part of phase one involves three days and the last four days of the week will then make up the second half. Each of these different halves will have their own purposes that you will need to follow to get the fullest effect of the entire diet. However, once you get past the first three days, the rest of it is so much easier.

The first half of phase one involves restricting your calories down to just 1000 per day. Yes, that is total, counting the green juice that you will be consuming. However, you will be restricting your diet even more than that as well. You must consume three green juices per day, and you are allowed one single sirtfood rich meal per day. That meal is usually going to be loaded with other veggies. Most people who quit this diet tend to do so at this point—the restrictions of calories for those first three days can be too much. However, remember that hunger is just that—hunger. You are not starving to death. It is temporary discomfort. When you can acknowledge that the hunger that you feel is just temporary, you will start seeing that at the end of the day, you can actually get great benefits. You will no longer be so intimidated by the idea of hunger, and getting through those days of caloric limitation will not seem so bad after all.

These first three days set your body up to function properly. Keep in mind that because most of your sustenance will be juice, you are probably going to be extra-hungry just due to the fact that you are not getting the fiber that would normally give you that staying power to keep your body happy and satiated. However, don't forget that it is only temporary and you will be just fine.

During the second half of phase one, you are actually allowed to raise your caloric content up significantly. During the second half of phase one, you will be allowed to eat up to 1500 calories per day. While this is still quite low if you are used to eating 2000+ calories per day, it is plenty for your body to function on. When you follow this diet with these limits, you will start seeing that you feel better and fuller. Getting to the second half of phase one will mean that everything is all downhill from there. You will be able to get through your diet so much easier when you have more food in your belly to keep you satisfied.

During these days, keep in mind that you should still be consuming green juice regularly. At this point in time, you are allowed to have two meals per day and the other two should be green juice. This will ensure that you are keeping your body working with that boosted metabolism while still guaranteeing that you have the deficit in calories that you need to keep losing weight. When you do so, you will start making great progress and seeing great strides as well.

Keep in mind that exercise must be maintained as normal during this phase of the diet. You want to ensure that you are creating as much of a calorie deficit as possible. This means making sure that you are getting those calories cut down where you can, such as through exercising to burn more, you will lose more weight as well. However, make sure that you are mindful of the limitations that you have. In particular, you may find that you start feeling dizzy or struggling in other ways, and because of this, you want to make sure that you pay close attention to how you feel along the way. This will ensure that you are carefully minding what you can do and what you cannot in hopes of avoiding injury. If you need to lighten up, especially during those first three days, then do so.

Phase Two

The second phase of this diet is the maintenance plan, and this part lasts two more weeks. The second phase is really just defined by the fact that you are looking to maintain a calorie deficit while still encouraging a high level of sirtuin consumption. By doing so, you will be able to continue burning off the weight. This stage is all about staying healthy but also is less restrictive than the previous phase.

When you get to the second phase of this diet, you are free to go back to eating three meals per day and a snack if you want to. There is no calorie limit during phase two, but it is still recommended that you maintain a good calorie deficit, and the best way for you to get that involves you eating only about 1500 calories per day. As you get through this diet, you will find yourself enjoying more foods as well.

Keep in mind that during the maintenance two weeks, you should still be enjoying your green juice daily, with at least one serving per day. This will help you to keep up those higher levels of sirtuins as you need to thrive. If you know what you are doing, you should be able to provide yourself with those added benefits and weight loss.

At this time, your sole purpose is to ensure that you are getting the right amount of calories and ensuring that at the end of the day, you also get the right amount of sirtuins to keep your body in that state of burning calories quickly enough to allow you to lose weight. Of course, you will not need to constantly stay in a state of deprivation—but until you are at the weight that you are happy with, you will need to do so.

Again, you want to keep up the exercise here to ensure that you are burning calories as well. You want to work to ensure that as you burn those calories, you will be able to lose weight. Over time, you will get to your desired weight. Keep in mind, however, that this phase officially only lasts for two weeks before it is over, and you will have to choose what you want to do afterward.

After Completing the Phases

After you have finished the two phases, you have a few more options on what you can do. You could simply decide that you are entirely finished with the diet and move on, choosing to do nothing more at all. This is perfectly fine, especially if you have decided that either this diet is not right for you or if you have decided that you lost the weight that you wanted. This is an entirely valid option. After all, this diet is not meant to last forever. You are well within your right to decide that you have finished up with it and are done.

Or, you could also choose to start the diet over, beginning right back at phase one. This way, you would re-trigger that state of metabolism to help yourself to lose weight quicker. If you need to do so, simply reverting right back to just 1000 calories per day is a great way to do so. From there, you would simply go through the phases again, spending three days at 1000 calories, then moving on as you did the first time.

You could also choose some sort of modified diet that you can use to help yourself to lose weight as well. You could, for example, stick to the phase two diet as well. After all, sticking to 1500 calories per day while exercising should still yield great weight loss efforts a swell over time. You will get those great benefits with ease so long as you are willing and able to go through the efforts.

What you choose to do is up to you, but remember that the foods that you will consume on this diet are meant to be healthy. They are some of the best foods on the planet that you can consume for your own health, and if at all possible, you should continue to consume them as much as possible. If you find that some of these recipes are particularly enjoyable, you might even choose to begin consuming them even more often as well, granting you all sorts of options to mix up your normal diet with great, healthy foods.

Tips and Tricks to Stick to Diets

When you want to start a diet, one of the most important things that you will need to remember is that you want to find ways to keep yourself on it. Diets, especially early on, can be difficult to follow just due to the fact that so much of what you eat whenever you are consuming foods is simply habitual. You consume foods that you do because you have taught yourself that you will do so. These become habits that can be hard to beat if you simply mindlessly follow them. You might be used to following these diets just due to the fact that you usually do, and because of that, trying to shift over to something as restrictive as the sirtfood diet seems impossible.

However, when you go into a diet with the right mindset, you can help yourself to stick to it. Knowing what to expect and why to expect it is crucial if you want to make progress. Knowing that you are going into a diet with the goal of losing weight and understanding what motivates you matters immensely and will ensure that at the end of the day, you are driven to do what you do. Let's go over some simple tips and tricks that you can implement that will help you to stick to any diet. Remember, it is all about the habits, and the sooner that you get those good habits into place, the sooner you will be able to ensure that you are successfully following your diet.

Stick to realistic expectations

Remember that you need to have realistic

expectations for any diet. This means that if you want to lose weight, you should have a realistic idea of just how much weight you are going to lose during your time trying to do so. If you want to lose 20 lbs., remember that won't happen overnight. You will have to spend weeks, or even months, working to lose that weight at a safe pace. After all, losing weight too quickly and your health can suffer. And, usually, people who pressure themselves to lose more weight than is really feasibly expectable tend to give up. By remembering to consider realistic expectations, you will help yourself to successfully get through your diet with much more ease. You won't feel disappointed or surprised about what happened, and you won't feel like you are failing if you don't see the number that you wanted to see immediately on the scale.

Remember your motivations

You could have all sorts of reasons you want to lose weight. Want to look good in your wedding dress? Trying to slim down so you can be ready for the summer? Are you interested in dropping the weight and getting healthier so that you can chase your children around without feeling like you are gasping for air? Think about what your motivations for getting healthier and losing weight are, even if you might think that they are "petty" or silly, and remember them when things get rough. By following along with the expectations that you set and remembering your motivations, it becomes easier to stick to your diet plan.

Avoid unhealthy foods

When you are shopping, cut out the junk food. While your diet may be yours alone, if you have all sorts of junk foods sitting around you, you are much more likely to dive in and oblige yourself than if you didn't have them. You want to make sure that you make it as easy as possible for you to stick to your diet, and that means making sure that you don't have junk foods within your sight, tempting you. If you have family members or roommates that insist on having those foods around, consider asking them to keep them put away somewhere that you then do not look. This will help you to stick to your diet because if it is out of sight, it is out of mind. It is easier to avoid temptation if the temptation isn't cookies sitting on the counter in front of you while you eat those carrot sticks.

Don't approach your diet as all or nothing

It can be easy to get caught up in the idea of all or nothing dieting. In this idea, you might think that because you had a few bites of junk food for the day, the day is lost, and you may as well indulge in more. Instead of doing so, you should instead consider working with yourself. Remind yourself that the day isn't lost just because you had a few treats. Instead of giving in or really indulging, simply move past your slip up and remind yourself that you can still make healthy choices for the rest of the day as well.

Prepare with healthy snacks

Sometimes, hunger strikes when you least expect it, and if you get hungry, you want to have something on hand that you can enjoy that will be healthy instead. Especially if you are out of the home often, preparing your snacks becomes even more important. This is because if you are hungry and have to buy something while out and about, you have an increased chance of it being unhealthy for you, which is highly problematic as well. You must ensure that you are choosing out foods that are healthy, and that means being ready with snacks when hunger strikes as well.

Practice mindful eating

When you shift over to mindful eating, you remind yourself that you can control your diet simply by focusing on the foods that you eat. Focus on the benefits of the foods that you consume. Pay attention to how they nourish your body and help you to grow stronger. Acknowledge how important those healthy choices are so that you can ensure that you are on the right track. When you eat those healthy foods mindfully, you will find that it is much easier to stick to your diet just because you are improving your relationship with the foods that you are eating.

Track your progress

As you work on your diet, make sure that you track the progress that you make. While you can't expect to see, the scale moves every single day, tracking your weight and your body's transformation over the time that your diet can actually help you to stick to your guns and keep yourself motivated for longer. This is because you will be able to track progress, even if it is not as much as you may have initially wanted to see.

Find an accountability buddy

If at all possible, follow the diet with someone that you know will stick to it with you. When you choose someone who is motivated to follow the same diet, you then have someone that you know will be able to help you out and keep you on track as well. This means that when it comes right down to it, you will stay on track and see better luck. If at all possible, get your family to stick to your diet. While you may not need to restrict the calories consumed for everyone else, you can still see great benefits in eating the same healthy dinners, and that can help you to feel less left out when you see everyone else eating as well. When you have other people making those healthy lifestyle changes, you will be more likely to stick to them as well.

Chapter 5: Green Drink Recipes

When you are following the sirtfood diet, one of the most important staples of all is the green juice that you must consume almost religiously. This juice is meant to provide you with the deliciousness of these various sirtfoods while also providing you with the nutritional value and the benefits that they will afford you. You will be consuming green juice daily during your time dieting, but after you have completed the two phases of this diet, it is recommended that you continue to drink the green juice regularly. Of course, you might decide to mix it up from time to time as well.

As you go through this chapter, we will begin with the classic sirtfood diet green juice recipe that will be your staple during the diet. However, we will also go over several other green juice and smoothie recipes that may appeal to you as well over time. Through mixing things up sometimes, you should find yourself enjoying all sorts of other flavors while still getting that nutritional burst.

Classic Sirtfood Green Juice

Ingredients:

- Kale (2 handfuls)
- Arugula (1 handful)
- Parsley (1 handful, preferably flat-leaf)
- Lovage (1 small handful—optional. *NOTE: Avoid lovage if pregnant)*
- Celery stalks (2 large—leaves attached)
- Green apple (1/2 of the apple)
- Lemon juice (1/2 a lemon's worth)
- Matcha powder (1 spoonful)

Instructions:

1. To begin, throw all of your greens together, tossing well. Then, add them to your juicer. If your juicer does not have the best results the first time, put the juice through a second time.
2. Throw your celery and apple into the juicer and allow the juice to be extracted.
3. Pour in your lemon juice and combine well. Add in matcha, mix well, and serve. Enjoy!

Tofu Green Smoothie

Ingredients:

- Banana (2, peeled and frozen)
- Kiwi (4, peeled and frozen)
- Mango (2 c. frozen)
- Silken tofu (12 oz.)
- Soy milk (2 c., unsweetened)
- Spinach (2 c., fresh baby variety)
- Turmeric (0.5 tsp)

Instructions:

1. Put all of your ingredients right into a blender and combine well. Serve chilled immediately.

Tropical Arugula Coconut Smoothie

Ingredients:

- Arugula (1 c.)
- Avocado (0.5)
- Coconut shreds (4 Tbsp.)
- Coconut water (0.33 c.)
- Lime (1/4 lime wedge, juiced and zested)
- Mango (0.5 c., frozen)

Instructions:

1. Put all of your ingredients right into your blender and combine well. Serve chilled immediately.

Matcha Smoothie

Ingredients:

- Almonds (2 Tbsp.)
- Banana (0.5 banana)
- Greek yogurt (0.25)
- Ice cubes (1 c.)
- Kale (0.5 c., fresh)
- Matcha powder (0.5 Tbsp.)
- Natural sweetener of choice (1 tsp)
- Soy milk (0.5 c.)
- Spinach (0.5 c.)

Instructions:

1. Put all of your ingredients right into your blender and combine well. Serve chilled immediately.

Note: _To thin, add extra milk. You can also thicken to the desired consistency by adding extra ice._

Strawberry-Arugula Smoothie

Ingredients:

- Arugula (2 oz.)
- Coconut water (14 oz.)
- Dates (5, pitted)
- Strawberries (5.5 oz., frozen)
- Watercress (1 oz.)

Instructions:

1. Put all of your ingredients right into your blender and combine well. Serve chilled immediately.

Gingery Green Juice

Ingredients:

- Celery stalks (5, trimmed)
- English cucumber (0.5)
- Ginger (1-inch stretch, peeled)
- Granny smith apple (1)
- Kale (1 bunch, roughly 5 oz.)
- Parsley (handful fresh)

Instructions:

1. Begin by prepping your veggies. Wash them up and cut them into chunks that will be manageable for your processer.
2. Juice, or blend on high. Enjoy!

Pineapple-Kale-Ginger Juice

Ingredients:

- Kale (1 c., chopped)
- Frozen pineapple (1 c., pieced)
- Ginger (1-inch piece, peeled)
- Cold water (1 c.)
- Ice cubes to taste

Instructions:

1. Put all ingredients into the blender and combine until liquefied and creamy. Add more ice if you prefer it to be thicker.

Grapefruit-Herb Juice

Ingredients:

- Basil (5 or 6 fresh sprigs)
- Cantaloupe (1/4 melon)
- Coconut sugar (1 Tbsp.)
- Cold water (1 c.)
- Cucumbers (2, peeled)
- Grapefruit (juice from 2)
- Mint (2 leaves)

Instructions:

1. Place all of the ingredients into a food processor and combine well until fully incorporated and smooth.
2. Put a strainer over a bowl and then put cheesecloth over the strainer.
3. Pour juice through the cheesecloth and strainer. Pick up the cloth and squeeze the pulp to get all juice out.
4. Serve immediately, or refrigerate and serve chilled later.

Celery-Pear Green Juice

Ingredients:

- Celery (2 stalks)
- Kale (3 c.)
- Mint (2 Tbsp., fresh)
- Pears (6, sliced with seeds removed)

Instructions:

1. Combine all ingredients through a juicer. Chill and serve.

Green Veggie Juice

Ingredients:

- Cucumbers (2)
- Celery (3-5 stalks)
- Broccoli stem (1 large, remove all florets before adding)
- Kale (2-3 leaves)
- Apple or pear (0.5, seeds removed)
- Ginger (1-2 inches, peeled)
- Lemon (0.5, peeled before juicing, or squeezing the juice into the cup at the end)

Instructions:

1. Prepare all of the ingredients, then cut small enough to fit into the juicer. Juice, then serve well over ice.

Chapter 6: Breakfasts

Breakfast is incredibly important. On this diet, sometimes, your breakfast will be a green juice drink, which is perfectly fine. However, other times, you will also be consuming other breakfasts as well, especially in phase two part of this diet. If you want to be able to enjoy a good, healthy, hearty meal on the sirtfood diet, then you are in the right place—keep reading through this chapter to get several delicious options that will keep you full and provide that sirtfood goodness that you need to succeed. Enjoy!

Strawberry Pancakes

Ingredients:

- Buckwheat flour (quarter c.)
- Chopped strawberries (4 oz.)
- Egg (1)
- Milk (1 c.)
- Olive oil (2 tsp)
- Orange juice (1 orange, fresh squeezed)

Instructions:

1. In a bowl, pour in the milk and mix with the egg and half of the olive oil. Sift your flour onto the milk and mix, making it creamy. Put it to the side.
2. Once rested for 15 minutes, prepare a frying pan by greasing with the rest of the oil and setting a burner to medium heat. Pour in your batter a quarter at a time.
3. Toss some strawberry bits onto the pancake batter before it sets on the frying pan. Flip after a few minutes and move onto a serving tray or individual plates. Repeat with the rest of your mixture.
4. When serving, pour a bit of orange juice over the pancakes.

Porridge with Walnuts

Ingredients:

- Chia seeds (1 tsp)
- Rolled oats (2 oz.)
- Soy milk (1 c.)
- Strawberries (3.5 oz.)
- Walnut halves (4, chopped)
- Water (3.5 oz.)

Instructions:

1. Pour all of the ingredients, except for the chia seeds, into a blender and process.
2. Toss in the chia seeds and mix them into the porridge. To have the porridge set, place the mixture into the fridge and chill.
3. When serving, top with walnuts.

<u>Strawberry Granola</u>

Ingredients:

- Almonds (3.5 oz., chopped)
- Buckwheat flakes (9 oz.)
- Dried strawberries (3.5 oz.)
- Ground cinnamon (1.5 tsp)
- Ground ginger (1.5 tsp)
- Honey (2 Tbsp.)
- Oats (7 oz.)
- Olive oil (quarter c.)
- Walnuts (3.5 oz., chopped)

Instructions:

1. Pour in cinnamon, both nuts, ginger, buckwheat flakes, and the oats into a bowl.
2. Warm up the honey and oil in a pan. Stir the honey while it melts.
3. Set your oven to 300° F. As your oven reaches baking temperature, take the honey oil, and pour it onto the other ingredients and mix thoroughly.
4. Spread the granola mixture onto a baking sheet (or a few depending on size) and toss it into the oven. Bake for 50 minutes.
5. Remove the granola from heat and allow it to cool. Mix in the dried strawberry and serve or store.

Chocolate Granola

Ingredients:

- Cacao powder (quarter c.)
- Chia seeds (2 Tbsp.)
- Coconut flakes (quarter c.)
- Coconut oil (2 Tbsp., melted)
- Dark chocolate (2 Tbsp.)
- Maple syrup (quarter c.)
- Rolled oats (2 c.)
- Salt
- Vanilla extract (half a tsp)

Instructions:

1. Preheat your oven to 300°. In a bowl, mix the vanilla extract, coconut oil, salt, maple syrup, and cacao powder.
2. Take a pan and heat on medium. Pour your mixture into the pan and cook until it thickens up. Remove from heat and set the syrup you just made aside.
3. Using another bowl, mix the chia seeds, oats, and coconut.
4. Add the syrup to this mixture and mix. Press the granola onto a baking sheet that is lined with parchment paper. Toss into the oven.
5. Bake for 35 minutes, remove from heat and allow the granola time to cool down completely. Crumble and serve or save for later.

Strawberry yogurt

Ingredients:

- Cocoa powder
- Plain Greek yogurt (3.5 oz.)
- Strawberries (2 oz., chopped)
- Walnut halves (6, chopped)

Instructions:

1. Take half of the strawberry bits you have chopped and toss it into the yogurt.
2. Stir in walnuts and mix.
3. Garnish with more walnut bits and cocoa powder.

Chocolate Waffles

Ingredients:

- Almond milk (2 c.)
- Baking powder (1 tsp)
- Baking soda (1 tsp)
- Buckwheat flour (1 c.)
- Cacao powder (half c.)
- Coconut oil (half c., melted)
- Dark brown sugar (quarter c.)
- Dark chocolate (2 oz., chopped)
- Eggs (2)
- Flaxseed meal (quarter c.)
- Lemon juice (1 Tbsp.)
- Salt
- Vanilla extract (2 tsp)

Instructions:

1. In a bowl, mix the lemon juice and almond milk. Let it rest for a couple of minutes.
2. In a separate bowl, toss in the salt, baking soda, baking powder, cacao powder, flaxseed meal, and buckwheat flour.
3. After the lemon juice and almond milk mixture has gotten a chance to sit, mix all of the ingredients together. It is strongly suggested to mix the liquid into the dry mixture first and stir gently. Do not over mix.

4. Pour the mixture into waffle iron and cook until golden brown. Repeat until there is no batter left. Serve and enjoy.

Blueberry Muffins

Ingredients:

- Almond milk (half c.)
- Arrowroot starch (quarter c.)
- Baking powder (1.5 tsp)
- Buckwheat flour (1 c.)
- Coconut oil (2 Tbsp., melted)
- Eggs (2)
- Fresh blueberries (1 c.)
- Maple syrup (2 Tbsp.)
- Salt

Instructions:

1. Preheat your oven to 350° F. Prepare a muffin tin by greasing it or using muffin liners.
2. In a bowl, toss in the baking powder, salt, buckwheat flour, and arrowroot starch.
3. In a separate bowl, whip together eggs, oil, milk, and syrup. Add in the dry mixture and fold in the fresh blueberries.
4. Pour the batter into the muffin tin and throw it in the oven. After baking for 25 minutes, remove the tin from heat and allow the muffins to cool before serving.

Salmon and Kale Omelet

Ingredients:

- Almond milk (2 Tbsp.)
- Eggs (6)
- Kale (2 c.)
- Olive oil (2 Tbsp.)
- Pepper
- Salt
- Scallions (4, chopped)
- Smoked salmon (4 oz.)

Instructions:

1. In a bowl, whip together the eggs, coconut milk, salt, and pepper. Set the mixture aside.
2. Heat up a pan with your oil. When hot, pour the egg mixture in. Allow the egg to cook undisturbed so it can begin to set.
3. Pour on the scallions, salmon, and kale on top and lower heat.
4. Cover the pan and let everything cook until the omelet is done, which should take roughly five minutes.
5. Remove the lid and cook for one more minute. Move to a plate, roll up, and serve.

Cheesy Eggs with Arugula

Ingredients:

- Arugula chopped (1 oz.)
- Eggs (4)
- Grated cheese (3 oz.)
- Ground turmeric (half tsp.)
- Olive oil (1 Tbsp.)
- Parsley (1 Tbsp.)

Instructions:

1. Grease four ramekins with your oil. Put a bit of arugula in each one.
2. Preheat your oven to 425° F. While your oven is heating up, creak an egg into each ramekin and sprinkle the parsley, turmeric, and cheese over it.
3. Toss in the ramekins into the oven and bake until the eggs are set. This should take roughly 15 minutes. Once the eggs have cooked through, remove from heat, and serve.

Poached Eggs and Arugula

Ingredients:

- Pepper
- Salt
- Olive oil (1 tsp)
- Fresh arugula (1 oz.)
- Eggs (2)

Instructions:

1. Wash your arugula leaves and spread them over a serving plate. Drizzle a bit of olive oil over the leaves.
2. Take a saucepan and place it on the stove. Pour some water in and bring it to a boil. Slowly pour in the eggs. Consider cracking the eggs one at a time into a ladle and using that to slowly introduce the eggs to the boiling water to avoid accidentally breaking the yokes. Allow the eggs to cook until the whites have set and cooked through.
3. Remove the eggs and place them on top of the arugula leaves. Add a pinch of salt and pepper to them and serve.

Twice Baked Potatoes

Ingredients:

- Butter (2 Tbsp.)
- Cheddar cheese (half c., shredded)
- Chives
- Cooked bacon (4 strips)
- Eggs (4)
- Pepper
- Russet Potatoes (4)
- Salt
- Sour cream (3 Tbsp.)

Instructions:

1. Prepare your oven by setting it to 400° F. Bake your potatoes for 45 minutes.
2. Remove the potatoes from heat and cut them lengthwise. Do not cut through them completely. Use a spoon to scoop out some of the potato flesh. Place the potato flesh into a bowl.
3. Add the sour cream and butter to the potato flesh and mix it until smooth.
4. Take the potato mixture and spoon it back inside the potato skins. Top with cheese, an egg, and a slice of bacon. Place the loaded potatoes into a baking sheet.
5. Reduce the heat on the oven to 375° F and place the baking sheet inside. Bake until the eggs have set.

6. Remove from heat and top with a bit more
cheese and freshly cut chives. Serve and enjoy.

Chapter 7: Lunches

On the days where you will be consuming a meal for lunch, you want to make sure that you have something that is wholesome and hearty. You want to feel like you have nourished your body greatly, and by following these sirtfood-dense recipes, you will do exactly that. Many of these meals can be made ahead of time as well to provide you with healthy meals without having to cook right when it is time to serve. Create large batches of some of these meals and serve them for several days for your own lunches to give yourself that beneficial boost to your diet that you want to get!

Moroccan Chicken Casserole

Ingredients:

- Bird's eye chili (1, chopped)
- Carrot (1, chopped)
- Chicken breasts (4, cubed)
- Chicken stock (1 pint)
- Coriander (2 Tbsp.)
- Corn flour (1 oz.)
- Dried apricots (6, halved)
- Ground cinnamon (1 tsp)
- Ground cumin (1 tsp)
- Ground turmeric (1 tsp)
- Medjool dates (4, halved)
- Red onion (1, sliced)
- Tinned chickpeas (9 oz.)
- Water (2 oz.)

Instructions:

1. Combine your cinnamon, stock, turmeric, cumin, chili, carrot, chickpeas, chicken, and onion in a pan.
2. Turn on the heat and bring your mixture to a boil. Once boiling, reduce heat and allow to simmer for 25 minutes.
3. Toss in the apricot and dates and simmer an additional ten minutes.
4. Mix the water and cornflour together. Pour the pasta into the pan and mix.

5. Add in the coriander and mix. Serve.

Coq Au Vin

Ingredients:

- Bacon (3.5 oz., chopped)
- Button mushrooms (1 lb.)
- Carrots (3, chopped)
- Chicken thighs (16)
- Garlic cloves (3, crushed)
- Garni (1 bouquet)
- Olive oil (2 Tbsp.)
- Parsley (3 Tbsp., chopped)
- Plain flour (2 Tbsp.)
- Red onions (2, chopped)
- Red wine (1.5 pints)

Instructions:

1. Take your chicken and coat it with flour.
2. Pour the oil into a pan and place over medium-high heat. Toss in your chicken and brown it on all sides. Set the chicken aside.
3. Preheat your oven to 350° F. While the oven is getting ready, using the same pan as before, cook your bacon with the red onion.
4. When the bacon is to your liking and the red onion is nice and soft, pour in the red wine and throw in the garlic, carrots, chicken, and the bouquet garni.
5. Toss everything into an oven-safe dish and place it in the oven. Bake for an hour.
6. Remove the bouquet garni and skim the fat.

7. Add in your mushrooms and parsley and bake
   an additional 15 minutes. Serve.

Chili Con Carne

Ingredients:

- Beef stock (14 oz.)
- Bird's eye chilies (2, chopped)
- Celery stick (1, chopped)
- Cocoa powder (1 Tbsp.)
- Cumin (1 Tbsp.)
- Garlic cloves (2, crushed)
- Kidney beans (7 oz.)
- Minced beef, lean (1 lb.)
- Olive oil (1 Tbsp.)
- Red onions (2, chopped)
- Red pepper (1, chopped)
- Red wine (6 oz.)
- Tomato puree (2 Tbsp.)
- Tomatoes (14 oz., chopped)
- Turmeric (1 Tbsp.)

Instructions:

1. Pour your oil into a pan and begin heating. Toss in the onion and cook until the onion is translucent and soft.
2. Toss in the cumin, chili, turmeric, garlic, and celery and continue cooking.
3. Add the meat and cook for five minutes. After this period of cooking, pour in the cocoa powder, red pepper, kidney beans, tomato puree, tomatoes, stock, and red wine. Allow

simmering on low heat, covered. Stir on occasion.
4. After roughly 45 minutes, the chili is ready to serve.

Chicken and Bean Casserole

Ingredients:

- Cannellini beans (14 oz.)
- Carrots (2, chopped)
- Celery sticks (4)
- Chicken stock (3 pints)
- Chicken thighs (8)
- Garlic clove (1, crushed)
- Mushrooms (4)
- Olive oil (1 Tbsp.)
- Red onions (2, chopped)
- Red peppers (2, chopped)
- Soy sauce (2 Tbsp.)
- Tomatoes (14 oz., chopped)

Instructions:

1. Get a skillet ready with your oil and place it over medium-high heat. Sauté your garlic and onions.
2. Once the onion has softened, toss in the chicken and cook for five minutes. Toss in the red peppers, celery, mushrooms, carrots, and cannellini beans.
3. Pour in the soy sauce, stock, and tomatoes and boil. Once boiling, reduce the heat and simmer.
4. Remove from heat after 45 minutes. Serve.

Prawn and Coconut Curry

Ingredients:

- Bird's eye chilies (2)
- Coconut milk (14 oz.)
- Coriander (1 oz., chopped)
- Garlic cloves (3, crushed)
- Ground coriander (half tsp)
- Lime (1, juice)
- Olive oil (1 Tbsp.)
- Red onion (3, chopped)
- Shelled prawns (14 oz.)
- Tomatoes (14 oz., chopped)
- Turmeric (half tsp)

Instructions:

1. In a blender, process the chilies, turmeric, ground coriander, lime juice, garlic, onions, and tomatoes. Process until your ingredients form a smooth paste.
2. Heat the oil in a pan and pour in the paste. Once thoroughly warmed, stir in the coconut milk. Toss in the prawns and cook until pink and cooked through.
3. Serve the curry over rice.

Spiced Lamb

Ingredients:

- Bird's eye chili (1, chopped)
- Garlic cloves (3, crushed)
- Ground cinnamon (quarter tsp)
- Ground coriander (half tsp)
- Ground cumin (1 tsp)
- Lamb shoulder (3 lb.)
- Olive oil (2 Tbsp.)
- Red onions (3, sliced)
- Turmeric (1 tsp)

Instructions:

1. In a bowl, mix a tablespoon of olive oil with garlic, chili, cinnamon, coriander, cumin, and turmeric. Place the lamb into the spice mixture and allow it to marinate for at least an hour.
2. Preheat your oven to 325° F. While your oven is getting ready, place the remaining tablespoon of oil on a pan and set it over medium-high heat. Sear the lamb shoulder on all sides.
3. Once seared, move the lamb shoulder onto an oven-safe dish and toss it in the oven. Bake for four hours.
4. When done, remove the lamb from heat and serve with your favorite sides.

Steak and Mushroom Noodles

Ingredients:

- Baby spinach leaves (3 oz., chopped)
- Chestnut mushrooms (3.5 oz., sliced)
- Fresh Cilantro (1 Tbsp.)
- Ginger (1 inch, chopped)
- Kale (3 oz., chopped)
- Miso paste (2 Tbsp.)
- Olive oil (2 Tbsp.)
- Red chili (1, sliced)
- Red onion (1, chopped)
- Shitake mushrooms (3.5 oz., halved)
- Sirloin steaks (2)
- Star anise (1)
- Udon noodles (5 oz.)
- Warm water (1.5 pints)

Instructions:

1. In a pan, toss in the ginger, miso paste, star anise, and water. Bring to a boil, then reduce heat to allow ingredients to simmer.
2. Following the instructions on the packaging, prepare the udon noodles, draining them, and setting aside.
3. Grease a pan and place over medium-high heat. Cook the steaks to your preferred level of doneness.

4. Grab the kale, spinach, mushrooms, and cilantro and toss them into the miso broth. Cook for five minutes.
5. Fry up the onion and chili in the pan you used to cook your steak. Oil lightly if needed. Cook until soft.
6. Place the noodles in serving bowls. Pour in the miso and veggies, and top with slices of steak.

Tofu Wraps

Ingredients:

- Any desired toppings, such as lettuce, kale, or tomato.
- Buckwheat (1 cup, processed until breadcrumb textured)
- Cornstarch (6 Tbsp.)
- Olive oil (2 Tbsp.)
- Oregano (1 tsp, dried)
- Paprika (half tsp)
- Soy milk (a third c.)
- Tofu (1 block, extra firm, pressed and drained)
- Whole wheat tortillas (6)

Instructions:

1. Preheat the oven to 425° F. Get a baking pan ready by blanketing it with parchment paper or greased aluminum foil.
2. Grab the tofu and cut it into 24 bite-sized cubes. Set aside.
3. In a bowl, mix the buckwheat crumbs, seasoning, and oil. Set aside.
4. Dip the tofu into cornstarch, then soy milk, then the buckwheat mixture, and finally place it on the baking sheet. Repeat this until all the tofu gets transferred onto the baking sheet. Try to give the tofu pieces space, so they crisp up.

5. Bake for 25 minutes. Remove from the oven and turn over all the tofu pieces. Continue to bake for another 10 minutes.
6. Remove from heat and put the tofu into tortilla wraps with your preferred toppings.

Kale and Chicken Curry.

Ingredients:

- Birds eye chili (1, minced)
- Boneless, skinless chicken thigh (1.5 cups, cut into bite-sized bits)
- Cardamom pod (1)
- Chicken stock (1 cup)
- Cilantro to garnish
- Curry powder (half Tbsp.)
- Garlic (2 cloves, crushed and minced)
- Ginger (half Tbsp.)
- Light coconut milk (a third of a cup, from a can for cooking, not for drinking)
- Olive oil (half Tbsp.)
- Red onion (1, diced)
- Tomato (1 c., chopped)
- Turmeric powder (1 Tbsp.)

Instructions:

1. Combine chicken, a teaspoon of oil, and a teaspoon of turmeric. Coat the chicken well and allow it to marinate as longs as you can.
2. Get a pan ready by greasing it and placing over medium-high heat. Cook the chicken until nicely browned. Set it aside.
3. Using the same pan, sauté garlic, onion, ginger, and chili with olive oil.

4. Toss in curry powder and 2 teaspoons of turmeric.
5. Add in coconut milk and tomato, along with cardamom pods and chicken stock. Lower the heat and simmer for half an hour.
6. Toss in the chicken you cooked earlier and throw in the kale. Cook until the kale wilts.
7. Serve with rice and garnish with cilantro.

Arugula and Kale Chicken Salad

Ingredients:

- Arugula (1 c., chopped)
- Buckwheat flour (an eighth of a c.)
- Chicken breast (1)
- Crushed red pepper
- Egg white (from 1 egg)
- Green onion (1, minced)
- Honey (1 tsp)
- Kale (2 c., chopped)
- Lemon juice (1 Tbsp.)
- Olive oil (2 Tbsp.)
- Parsley (half tsp, dried)
- Salt and pepper
- Tomato (half c., diced)
- Walnuts (quarter c., ground)

Instructions:

1. Get your oven ready for baking by setting it to 375° F. In the meantime, get a baking sheet and either lightly grease it with oil or blanket it with a piece of parchment paper.
2. Get your chicken breast seasoned with salt and pepper on both sides. How much depends on your individual palate.
3. Crack your egg into a small dish. Remove the yoke, or when cracking open the egg, use its

own shell to keep the yoke separated, to begin with.

4. Combine the buckwheat flour with the crushed red pepper, walnuts, and parsley.

5. Take the chicken breast and dip it in the egg white, coating it completely, then dip it into the flour.

6. Spray the chicken with olive oil and place it on the baking tray. Bake for 20 minutes.

7. Remove the chicken from heat and place it on a cutting board. Slice it up into strips or into cubes; it is your choice here.

8. Mix the lemon juice, honey, and onion with two tablespoons of olive oil.

9. In a large bowl, toss the arugula, tomato, and kale. Pour in the dressing you made and toss it some more, coating it evenly throughout. Serve the salad topped with bits of chicken breast and enjoy.

Goat Cheese Pizza

Ingredients:
For the crust

- Buckwheat flour (8 oz.)
- Dried yeast (2 tsp)
- Olive oil (1 tsp)
- Salt
- Water (5 oz.)

For the topping

- Arugula leaves (1 oz., chopped)
- Crumbled feta cheese (3 oz.)
- Passata (3 oz.)
- Red onion (1, chopped)
- Tomato (1, sliced)

Instructions:

1. Preheat your oven to 400° F. As you're waiting for your oven to get ready, grab a bowl and combine the pizza dough ingredients. Once thoroughly mixed, allow it to sit for an hour, doubling in size.
2. Take the dough and roll it out until you get your preferred crust thickness and size. Pour the passata and spread it over the pizza dough. Spread your toppings over the tomato sauce.

3. Stick the pizza in the oven and bake until the crust has browned and crisps. The cheese should also be melted.
4. Remove from heat and serve.

Chapter 8: Dinners

We usually spend dinners around the table at home with our families. Dinner becomes a sort of ritual in which we all get together and reconnect with our families. For this reason, it was a priority to design the dinners provided in this chapter around the family. These are meals that should be family-friendly for most people, though you may need to cut the spiciness levels of some dishes. Nevertheless, these recipes should give you that chance to reconnect with the people around you, gaining the benefit of being able to enjoy your time together. As you go through these recipes, give them a shot, and make enough to share with the whole family. You are bound to get some thumbs up around the table! Enjoy!

Asian Hotpot

Ingredients:

- Bean sprouts (50 g)
- Broccoli (50 g. chopped)
- Carrot (half, peeled, and cut)
- Chicken broth (500 ml)
- Cilantro (1 handful)
- Ginger sushi (20 g, chopped)
- Juice from half a lime
- Miso paste (1 Tbsp.)
- Parsley (1 handful, chopped)
- Raw tiger prawns (100 g)
- Rice noodles (50 g)
- Star anise (1, crushed)
- Tofu (100 g, chopped)
- Tomato puree (1 tsp)
- Water chestnuts (50 g)

Instructions:

1. Take a skillet and pour in your chicken stock, cilantro, lime juice, parsley, tomato puree, and star anise. Have everything simmer for ten minutes.
2. Toss in the water chestnuts, tofu, noodles, prawns, cabbage, and broccoli. Continue cooking until the prawns are cooked through.

3. Remove from heat and whisk in your miso paste and ginger sushi. When serving, garnish with parsley and fresh cilantro.

Lentil Soup

Ingredients:

- Bird's eye chili (half of one)
- Carrots (2, chopped)
- Celery sticks (2, chopped)
- Coriander (1 tsp, ground)
- Cumin (1 tsp, ground)
- Garlic clove (1, chopped)
- Olive oil (2 Tbsp.)
- Red lentils (6 oz.)
- Red onion (1, chopped)
- Salt and pepper
- Turmeric (1 tsp, ground)
- Vegetable stock (2 pints)

Instructions:

1. Pour your oil into a pan and place it over medium heat. When hot, throw in the onion and cook until translucent.
2. Add the garlic, cumin, turmeric, coriander, celery, chili, carrots, and lentils into the skillet and let it all cook through.
3. Pour in the vegetable broth and bring everything to a boil. Once boiling, lower the heat and allow the soup to simmer for 45 minutes.

4. If you want a smoother consistency, pour the
    soup into a food processor or blender and pulse
    until you get your preferred texture.
5. When serving, sprinkle a bit of salt and pepper.

<u>Turmeric Baked Salmon</u>

Ingredients:

- Birds eye chili (1, minced)
- Canned green lentils (third c.)
- Celery (1.5 cups, chopped)
- Chicken stock (half c.)
- Curry powder (1 tsp)
- Garlic (1 clove, minced)
- Lemon juice (quarter lemon)
- Olive oil (1 tsp)
- Parsley (1 Tbsp. chopped)
- Red onion (half c., diced)
- Salmon (4 oz., skinned)
- Tomatoes (1.5, diced)
- Turmeric powder (1 tsp)

Instructions:

1. Get your oven ready by preheating to 400° F.
2. On a medium-low flame, place olive oil in your frying pan and wait until the oil begins to shimmer. Put the garlic, onion, ginger, celery, and chili into the mixture. For 2-3 minutes, cook gently until it has started to soften. Apply the curry powder and cook for an additional minute.
3. Add the tomatoes and the stock, and then the lentils. Cook at a low temperature and boil for

10 minutes. Test the celery texture to decide if it is properly cooked for you.

4. Combine the turmeric, lemon juice, and oil in a small jar to make a sauce. Rub all the salmon on top and place the salmon on the baking tray. Cook until it starts to flake, for 10 minutes.

5. Top with parsley to serve.

Prawn Stir Fry

Ingredients:

- Birds eye chili (4)
- Buckwheat noodles (10 oz.)
- Celery (one and a third c., chopped)
- Chicken stock (2 c.)
- Garlic (4 cloves)
- Ginger (4 tsp. minced)
- Green beans (2 c., chopped)
- Kale (3 c., chopped)
- Olive oil (8 Tbsp.)
- Red onion (two-thirds c., diced)
- Shelled prawns (4 c.)
- Soy sauce (8 Tbsp.)

Instructions:

1. Heat up the frying pan. Cook the prawns with half of the oil and soy sauce. Three minutes to cook and cut the prawns.
2. Clean the pan for later with a paper towel.
3. Cook noodles according to their packaging and set aside.
4. Return the oil to the frying pan and add all the vegetables. Cook on medium-high heat for 2-3 minutes. Add stock then.
5. Bring the stock to the boiling point, then lower the temperature, allowing 2 minutes to simmer. Add the noodles and prawns. Bring to

a boil for a minute again before cooling off and
serving.

Prawn Arrabbiata

Ingredients:

- Birds eye chili (4, chopped finely)
- Buckwheat noodles (10 oz.)
- Canned crushed tomatoes (4 c.)
- Celery (1 c., diced)
- Garlic (4 cloves, minced)
- Olive oil (4 Tbsp.)
- Parsley (4 Tbsp., chopped)
- Red onions (1.5, chopped finely)
- Shrimp (1 lb., raw and shelled)
- White wine (8 Tbsp.)

Instructions:

1. Start by sautéing the onions, celery, and chili for two minutes in 4 tablespoons of olive oil. Then, increase the temperature to medium for another minute and let it simmer. Stir in the tomatoes and cook for about 30 minutes.
2. Prepare the spaghetti, following the box instructions. Strain the water and toss the olive oil with a tablespoon.
3. Apply the prawns to the sauce and cook, until finished but not overcooked, for 4 minutes. Add the spaghetti and parsley. Mix gently and serve.

Chicken Zucchini Stir Fry

Ingredients:

- Broth (1 c., chicken or veggie)
- Chicken breast (1 lb., thinly sliced)
- Corn starch (1 Tbsp.)
- Ginger (1 Tbsp., minced)
- Green onions (chopped to garnish)
- Honey (1 Tbsp.)
- Mirin (2 Tbsp.)
- Olive oil (1 Tbsp.)
  Garlic (1 Tbsp., minced)
- Sesame oil (2 tsp)
- Soy sauce (quarter c.)
- Zucchini (2 c., cut into thin half-circles)

Instructions:

1. In one dish, combine the soy sauce, broth, sugar, mirin, sesame oil, and corn starch and blend thoroughly.
2. Take a large saucepan and warm 1 tsp of medium-high olive oil. Cook half of the chicken in flat layers at a time. It should take about2-3 minutes per side.
3. After removing the chicken, throw in the last tsp of oil. Then add the garlic and ginger and simmer until it begins to smell good. Stir in the prepared sauce and set it aside. Whisk well as it warms and thickens for a minute.

4. Add the zucchini to the sauce and cook until
    tender, but allow it to keep some of its bite,
    normally only a few minutes. Take it off the fire
    and mix the chicken with the sauce. Top with
    green onions to serve.

Slow Cooker Vegetarian Curry

Ingredients:

- Carrots (4)
- Celtic sea salt
- Chili powder (quarter tsp.)
- Cinnamon (1 inch)
- Curry powder (2 Tbsp.)
- Garlic cloves (3)
- Onion (1)
- Sweet peas (250 g.)
- Sweet potatoes (2)
- Tapioca flour (2 Tbsp.)
- Tomato cubes (400 g)
- Vegetable broth (100 ml.)

Instructions:

1. Begin by chopping up the vegetables and potatoes. Take the garlic and mince it or push it through a press. Halve the peas. Take the onions, carrots, and sweet potatoes and toss them into the slow cooker.
2. Using a small bowl, mix your salt, cinnamon, chili powder, curry powder, tapioca flour, and cumin. Sprinkle this mixture onto your vegetables. Pour the vegetable broth over everything.
3. Cover the slow cooker and let it simmer at the low setting for six hours.

4. Stake the peas and tomatoes and stir them into the slow cooker. Cook for another hour at the low setting.
5. Serve. Consider serving with a side of cauliflower rice.

Spiced Chicken Cauliflower Couscous

Ingredients:

- Birds eye chili (1, diced)
- Capers (1 Tbsp.)
- Carrots (quarter c., diced)
- Cauliflower (1.5 c., riced)
- Chicken breast (1)
- Garlic (1 clove, minced)
- Ginger (1 tsp, minced)
  Olive oil (2 Tbsp.)
- Lemon juice (from half a lemon)
- Parsley (10 sprigs, chopped)
- Red onions (quarter c., diced)
- Sun-dried tomatoes (quarter c.)
- Turmeric powder (2 tsp)

Instructions:

1. Take your cauliflower and chop the florets into chunks. Toss these chunks into a food processor and blend until the cauliflower turns into little bits of "rice."
2. In a pan, sauté onions, chili, ginger, and garlic. Use a tablespoon of olive oil and cook over medium-high heat.
3. Pour in the turmeric and toss in the carrots and cauliflower. Cook for roughly three minutes.

4. Remove the mixture from heat and set off to
   the side. Stir in tomatoes and parsley.
5. Using the rest of your oil, cook the chicken over
   medium heat until cooked through. Add in the
   lemon juice, capers, and water. After a minute
   or two, toss in the cauliflower rice and sauce.
   Mix and serve. Garnish with cilantro.

Lemon Garlic Salmon

Ingredients:

- Dill (2 Tbsp., fresh and chopped)
- Garlic (8 cloves, crushed and minced)
- Lemon juice (third c., fresh)
- Olive oil (2 tsp)
- Pepper (a pinch)
- Salmon (4 pieces, skin attached)
- Salt (a pinch)

Instructions:

1. Begin by sprinkling salt and pepper onto the salmon. How much is entirely up to you.
2. Take a large skillet and warm your oil. When the oil is shimmering, place the salmon in the pan with the skin facing up. Cook for about four minutes. Flip the salmon so the skin is face down and sear.
3. Move the salmon to one side of the pan and squeeze in lemon juice and throw in your garlic. Sauté for a minute, basting the salmon with lemon juice in the meantime.
4. Stop cooking when the fish is cooked through and flakes easily. When serving, garnish with fresh dill.

Miso Tofu Stir Fry

Ingredients:

- Birds eye chili (2, diced)
- Brown miso paste (2 Tbsp.)
- Buckwheat noodles (half c.)
- Celery (1 stalk, finely chopped)
- Garlic (2 cloves, minced)
- Kale (1.25 c., ribs removed)
- Olive oil (4 tsp)
- Red onion (1, sliced in thin strips)
- Sesame seeds (4 tsp)
- Soy sauce (2 tsp)
- Tofu (1 package)
- Turmeric powder (2 tsp)
- Water (1 c.)
- White wine (2 Tbsp.)
- Zucchini (1, sliced into thin half-circles)

Instructions:

1. Get started by preparing a baking sheet. Line it with parchment paper or blanket it with aluminum foil. Preheat the oven to 400° in the meantime.
2. Take the miso paste and mix with your wine. Set the mixture off to the side. Cut your tofu into triangles and marinate it in the wine mixture.
3. Steam the kale, pulling it off the heat when it starts to wilt.

4. Slice up all of the vegetables and set to the side.
5. Place the tofu onto the baking sheet you prepared and cover with sesame seeds. Bake for twenty minutes, stopping early if the surface starts to caramelize.
6. Using the package instructions, make your buckwheat noodles.
7. When there are only five minutes left for the baking tofu, add olive oil to a frying pan and sauté the vegetables.
8. Serve the vegetables with the buckwheat noodles.

Sesame Chicken Salad

Ingredients:

- Baby kale (10 g)
- Chicken (150 g, shredded)
- Cucumber (1, sliced)
- Pak choi (60 g)
- Parsley (20 g, chopped)
- Red onion (half, sliced)
- Sesame seeds (1 tbsp.)

For the dressing

- Clear honey (1 tsp)
- Lime (1)
- Olive oil (1 Tbsp.)
- Sesame oil (1 tsp)
- Soy sauce (2 tsp)

Instructions:

1. Begin by taking out a skillet and brown the sesame seeds dry. Once properly browned, move the seeds to a plate and set them aside.
2. In a small container, pour in the lime juice, soy sauce, oils, and honey. Mix to create your salad dressing.
3. In a big bowl, toss in the red onion, pak choi, kale, cucumber, and parsley. Drizzle dressing on top.

4. Split the salad between two plates and top
   them with chicken. Sprinkle on sesame seeds
   and serve.

Chicken and Kale Curry

Ingredients:

- Olive oil (3 Tbsp.)
- Cinnamon (1 stick)
- Cardamoms (2, whole)
- Cloves (2, whole)
- Fennel seed (quarter tsp)
- Coriander powder (4 tsp)
- Cayenne powder (1 tsp)
- Turmeric (half tsp)
- Kale (4 leaves, chopped and de-stemmed)
- Chicken thighs (4, no skin or bones, cubed)
- Red onion (2 c., chopped)
- Garlic cloves (4, crushed and minced)
- Ginger (1 tsp)
- Tomato (1 c., chopped)
- Coconut milk (half c., canned)
- Water (1 c.)
- Salt

Instructions:

1. Prepare an instant pot by placing it on the sauté setting. Pour in olive oil and the whole spices. After a few minutes, toss in the ginger, onion, and garlic.
2. Once the onions are translucent, add the tomato, powdered spices, and coriander. Sauté

until the tomatoes have softened, stirring
regularly.
3. Turn off the instant pot and throw in the
chicken, water, coconut milk, salt, and kale.
Manually set the cooking time to five minutes
and seal.
4. Once the five minutes are over, change the
setting to warm and cook for an additional four
minutes. Open the release vent and then
quickly release the pressure.
5. Taste the curry and adjust the seasoning as you
see fit. Serve this over some rice or with
buckwheat noodles.

Chapter 9: Treats and Snacks

Just because you are on a diet doesn't mean that you can't enjoy treats sometimes or that you can't have a snack every now and then. By choosing recipes from this chapter, however, you can rest assured, knowing that whatever you have chosen to eat for yourself is going to be healthy and beneficial to you. You just need to pick out the foods and commit to enjoying them! Give them a shot and be surprised by just how much you enjoy the taste of being healthy! These foods are delicious, and you are going to wind up loving the additions to your diet that will also help you to lose weight along the way.

<u>*Truffles*</u>

Ingredients:

- Cocoa powder (2 Tbsp.)
- Coconut oil (1 Tbsp.)
- Hazelnuts (2 oz., chopped)
- Medjool dates (4)
- Shredded coconut (5 oz.)
- Walnuts (2 oz., chopped)

Instructions:

1. Pour the coconut oil, Medjool dates, cocoa powder, hazelnuts, walnuts, and shredded coconut into a blender. Cover with the lid and process everything until you have a creamy and smooth mixture.
2. Take a teaspoon and scoop up the truffle mix and roll it into a ball. Repeat until you are out of truffle mix.
3. Take the truffle balls and place them onto a parchment covered tray. Cover them and allow them to chill for an hour in the fridge.

No-Bake Pancakes

Ingredients:

- Cocoa powder (2 Tbsp.)
- Coconut oil (1 Tbsp.)
- Dates (4 oz.)
- Porridge oats (3 oz.)
- Strawberries (2 oz.)
- Unsalted peanuts (2 oz.)
- Walnuts (2 oz.)

Instructions:

1. Pour the cocoa powder, coconut oil, nuts, fruit, and oats into a blender. You should end up with a nice, thick mixture.
2. Take a baking sheet or use a flat surface and spread the pancake mixture. Press it to flatten and smoothen the texture.
3. Using a sharp knife, cut the mixture into even pieces. Garnish with additional cocoa powder or some shredded coconut flakes and enjoy.

Strawberry Yogurt

Ingredients:

- Fresh squeezed orange juice (1 orange)
- Honey (1 Tbsp.)
- Plain yogurt (16 oz.)
- Strawberries (6 oz.)

Instructions:

1. Freshly squeeze the juice out of your orange and pour it into a blender. Take your strawberries and, after giving them a quick rinse, toss them into the blender to join the orange juice. Pulse until smooth. Either use the fruit mixture as-is or run it through a fine sieve to remove the seeds and any additional fiber. Your choice here.
2. Place the fruit mix into a bowl and spoon in the yogurt and honey. Place everything into an ice cream maker and follow the directions on making yogurt.
3. Since not everyone has an ice cream maker, take the mixture and place it in the freezer for an hour. Pull it out afterward and whisk it around with a fork. Place it back in the freezer for an additional two hours and enjoy.

Walnut and Date Loaf

Ingredients:

- Baking soda (1 tsp)
- Banana (1, mashed)
- Eggs (3)
- Medjool dates (4 oz., chopped)
- Milk (8 oz.)
- Self-rising flour (9 oz.)
- Walnuts (2 oz., chopped)

Instructions:

1. Pull out a bowl and run the flour and baking soda through a sieve. Once you are done with that messy endeavor, combine your milk, dates, eggs, and banana. Combine well.
2. This recipe works best when you set your oven to 360° F. Preheat the oven prepare a loaf tin with some cooking spray or oil. Move the loaf mix into the loaf tin and smooth it down.
3. Place the tin into the oven and bake it for 45 minutes. Once time has passed, test the loaf with a fork or a prong and see if it comes out clean. If so, your bread is done. If not, bake for a few minutes more. When fully baked through, move the bread onto a wire rack and allow it to cool before serving.

Chocolate Brownies

Ingredients:

- Baking soda (half a tsp)
- Coconut oil (1 oz., melted)
- Dark chocolate (7 oz.)
- Eggs (3)
- Medjool dates (7 oz.)
- Vanilla extract (2 tsp)
- Walnuts (3.5 oz., chopped)

Instructions:

1. This recipe is meant to be baked at 350° F, so preheat your oven appropriately. While waiting for the oven to get up to temp, pour the vanilla extract, coconut oil, baking soda, eggs, dates, and chocolate into a food processor or blender.
2. Pulse until all the ingredients are nice and smooth. Toss in the walnuts and pulse quickly to mix them in.
3. Take a baking sheet and line it with parchment paper or grease it with a bit of oil. Pour the brownie mix onto the tray and place it into the oven.
4. Bake for 20 minutes or until baked to your liking.
5. Remove the tray from heat and allow it to cool. Slice the brownies and serve.

Kale Pizza Chips

Ingredients:

- Almonds (2 oz., ground)
- Kale (9 oz., chopped)
- Mixed herbs (half a tsp)
- Olive oil (2 Tbsp.)
- Onion powder (half a tsp)
- Oregano (half a tsp)
- Parmesan cheese (2 oz.)
- Tomato puree (3 Tbsp.)
- Water (3.5 oz.)

Instructions:

1. Get your oven ready by preheating to 325° F. Place the water, oil, onion powder, oregano, herbs, puree, cheese, and almonds into a blender and process as smoothly as you can.
2. Now throw the kale leaves into the mixture and coat them thoroughly. Place the kale leaves onto a baking sheet that's covered in parchment paper or lightly greased.
3. Move the sheet into the oven and bake for 15 minutes. They should come out nice and crispy.

Zucchini Bites

Ingredients:

- Zucchini (1 c., shredded and packed)
- Egg (1)
- Italian cheese blend (a third c.)
- Rice cereal (quarter c., crushed)
- Italian seasoning (three-quarters tsp)
- Garlic powder (quarter tsp)
- Salt and pepper

Instructions:

1. Prepare your oven by setting it to 400° F. While the oven is preheating, take your shredded zucchini and dry it out by placing it in a couple of paper towels and squeezing it to remove the excess liquid. Try to get as much out as possible as it will help the snacks crisp up in the oven.
2. Mix the zucchini shreds with the egg, cheese, cereal, and seasonings.
3. Get a baking sheet ready by placing parchment paper on it or grease it lightly with oil.
4. Take roughly two teaspoons of the zucchini mixture at a time and create little nuggets or balls. Place the zucchini bites onto the baking tray you prepared and move them into the oven. Bake for 25 minutes, flipping them halfway through.

5. Remove from heat and allow them to cool
slightly before serving.

Cheesy Vegan Kale Chips

Ingredients:

- Kale (4 bunches)
- Lemon juice (2 Tbsp.)
- Nutritional yeast (half c.)
- Sea salt
- Sunflower seeds (2 c.)
- Turmeric powder (1 tsp)
- Water (quarter c.)

Instructions:

1. To get this recipe right, you are going to need to prepare you sunflower seeds ahead of time. Take your seeds and soak them in water overnight. In the morning, or when you are ready to cook, drain the seeds and toss them into a blender or food processer. Pour in the lemon juice, turmeric, and yeast. Finally, pour in the quarter cup of water and blend everything together. If the mixture is too thick, try adding a bit more water.
2. Prepare your oven at 225° F. While the oven is preheating, take the kale and tear it up into small pieces, taking care to remove the pieces of stem.
3. When you are done with your kale, mix it into the sunflower batter and coat well.

4. Prepare a baking sheet with parchment paper or greasy it lightly. Place the pieces of kale on top in a single layer and bake for 40 minutes. Halfway through baking, flip the chips to ensure even crisping.

Coffee Nibbles

Ingredients:

- Almonds (half c.)
- Chia seeds (half Tbsp.)
- Dark chocolate cocoa powder (2 Tbsp.)
- Espresso (quarter c., cold)
- Medjool dates (4, pitted)
- Salt

Instructions:

1. Begin by soaking your dates in the espresso for half an hour. Remove the dates and save the coffee for a future step.
2. Place the coffee-soaked dates into a blender or food processor and pulse until you are left with a smooth puree. Pour in some of the coffee you saved to make a thick paste. Remember to start with less and add in more as needed. You can always add more liquid, but you will not be able to easily remove excess liquid.
3. Toss in the almonds, chia seeds, salt (just a bit will do), and cocoa powder into the food processor and pulse. You should end up with a chocolatey dough.
4. Grab your dough and form it into small, bite-sized balls. Place them on a tray or dish and refrigerate them to set.

Spiced Apples

Ingredients:

- Apples (4)
- Cinnamon sticks (2)
- Green tea (half a pint)
- Honey (2 Tbsp.)
- Star anise (4)

Instructions:

1. Grab the premade (or homemade, if you want this to be extra tasty) green tea and honey and pour them into a pan. Bring the mixture to a boil.
2. Once boiling, toss in the cinnamon, apples, and star anise.
3. Reduce the heat and allow everything to simmer for 15 minutes. Once the time is up, remove the apples and serve. Consider topping your apples with some yogurt.

Nutty Vegetable Bread

Ingredients:

- Bird's eye chili (1, chopped)
- Carrot (1, chopped)
- Celery stalks (3, chopped)
- Egg (1, whipped)
- Garlic (2 cloves, chopped)
- Haricot beans (3.5 oz.)
- Mushrooms (6 oz., chopped)
- Olive oil (2 Tbsp.)
- Parsley (2 Tbsp., chopped)
- Peanuts (3.5 oz., chopped)
- Red onion (1, chopped)
- Red wine (2 oz.)
- Turmeric powder (2 tsp)
- Walnuts (3.5 oz., chopped)
- Water (3.5 oz.)

Instructions:

1. Pour a bit of oil into a skillet and place over medium heat. When the oil is ready, toss in your turmeric, onion, mushrooms, celery, carrot, garlic, and chili. Cook until your vegetables have softened.
2. While the vegetables are cooking, set your oven to 375° F. Set the skillet aside after everything has softened.
3. Now focus on placing the haricot beans into a bowl and mix them with water, parsley, red

wine, egg, soy sauce, and nuts. Place the veggie mixture inside as well and continue to mix.

4. Grab a bread loaf tin and grease it with oil lightly or spray it with cooking spray. Pour the batter into the tin, making a nice even layer on top. Place the bread tin into the oven and bake for an hour.

5. Once time has been reached, check the bread with a fork or a skewer and see if any uncooked dough clings on. If not, the bread is done and needs to be removed from the oven. Allow the bread to sit for 15 minutes in the tin before trying to pull it out. Place the bread on a wire rack to allow it to cool completely before serving.

Chapter 10: A 2-Week Meal Plan

Congratulations! You've made it through the book and all the way to the end. At this point, you have seen what this book has to offer. You've seen several delicious recipes that are meant to keep you full and nourished. You've been provided with all sorts of ample opportunities to ensure that you are getting all of the good foods that you will need.

Creating your own meal plan is simple—all you will have to do is fill in the breakfasts, lunches, and dinners that you want to enjoy. What can really help for you would be working to give yourself very specific meals that work well with your specific schedule. If you know that Monday is going to be very busy for you, for example, you might want to have a slow cooker dinner prepared so you know that you have something that will be waiting for you when you get home. By making sure that you do this, you will be providing yourself with a better likelihood of giving yourself exactly what you want.

Having schedules will help you to stick to your meal plan that you create, and having a solid meal plan will help you to stick to your diet as well. The meal plan is your secret to dieting success—knowing what it will take is going to help you immensely, and all you have to do is know how to set it up. As you read through this chapter, you are being given a quick dieting meal plan that will show you what you can expect on the sirtfood diet. This is what you can expect to see for two weeks of the sirtfood diet, and by following this template, you will find that you can get the success that you are looking for. Before you know it, you will realize that success on this diet is easier than you thought.

PHASE ONE PART ONE

This first phase requires you to eat just 1000 calories per day. And in addition to this, you will be replacing three meals per day with green juice. This means that you can enjoy one meal per day. In this meal plan, you will be eating dinner each day, allowing you to enjoy the last meal of your day with your family at the dinner table. Keep in mind that you want to follow this limitation closely, and you want to also avoid any addition of red wine in those first few days. Of course, when you create your own meal plan, you can make your own adaptations. You could choose to eat a solid breakfast, or a lunch, or you could change up the meals in the dinner spot each day as well. Choose out whichever dietary choices sound the most appealing to you, so long as you follow the three juices per day.

Day 1

Breakfast: Green juice
Lunch: Green juice
Dinner: Asian hotpot
Snack: Green juice

Day 2

Breakfast: Green juice
Lunch: Green juice
Dinner: Miso tofu stir fry
Snack: Green juice

Day 3

Breakfast: Green juice
Lunch: Green juice
Dinner: Lemon garlicky salmon
Snack: Green juice

PHASE ONE PART TWO

The second part of the first phase of this diet is all about eating a bit more. Now, instead of just one meal per day, you are allowed to eat 1500 calories and two meals. Pick wisely. In this meal plan, you will see that you are instructed to eat any two meals each day, as well as two green juices per day, with the remaining meal of the day being replaced with a green juice as well. As before, you are free to make alterations. If you prefer breakfast and lunch, then go for it—just make sure that you are getting two meals per day and drinking two green juices per day to follow this part of your diet for the best results.

Day 4

Breakfast: Blueberry muffins

Lunch: Green juice
Dinner: Chicken zucchini stir fry
Snack: Green juice

Day 5

Breakfast: Green juice
Lunch: Tofu wraps
Dinner: Prawn stir fry
Snack: Green juice

Day 6

Breakfast: Strawberry pancakes
Lunch: Green juice
Dinner: Prawn arrabbiata
Snack: Green juice

Day 7

Breakfast: Green juice
Lunch: Chili con carne
Dinner: Sesame chicken salad
Snack: Green juice

PHASE TWO: MAINTENANCE

After getting this far in your diet, you are officially in maintenance mode. This phase involves you working to keep up with your diet while also giving you more freedom to consume what you want when you want it.

At this point, you are free to consume as much as you want throughout the day, so long as you are keeping that 1500 calorie limit and while also keeping in at least one green juice per day as well. This means that you must be mindful of your portions so that you can be certain you are getting what you need for your diet. Get creative! Enjoy the meals that you have available to you in this cookbook! If you can do so, you are likely to make great progress. All you have to do is ensure that you enjoy the foods in front of you. In this meal plan, you will see that the green juice is automatically included with breakfast each day. Of course, you can change it up; however you would like to ensure that you enjoy your diet that you are on.

Day 8

Breakfast: Porridge with walnuts, green juice
Lunch: Moroccan chicken casserole
Dinner: Turmeric baked salmon

Day 9

Breakfast: Salmon and kale omelet, green juice
Lunch: Spiced lamb
Dinner: Slow cooker vegetarian curry

Day 10

Breakfast: Chocolate waffles, green juice
Lunch: Goat cheese pizza

Dinner: Lemon garlic salmon

Day 11

Breakfast: Chocolate granola, green juice
Lunch: Chicken and bean casserole
Dinner: Spiced chicken cauliflower couscous

Day 12

Breakfast: Strawberry yogurt, green juice
Lunch: Coq au vin
Dinner: Asian hotpot

Day 13

Breakfast: blueberry muffins, green juice
Lunch: Kale chicken curry
Dinner: Turmeric baked salmon

Day 14

Breakfast: Poached eggs and arugula, green juice
Lunch: Spiced lamb
Dinner: Prawn stir fry

Conclusion

And, that concludes this book! Congratulations! You've made it all the way through. Arguably, you have taken the most important step toward the success that you need—you have taken the first one. That first step, recognizing that you want to commit to a diet enough that you have taken the time to read through an entire book, is incredibly telling—it shows that you are driven and that you are ready to lose the weight. You just have to find a way to make it happen, and that is exactly what this book was here to give you.

No matter whether your intention is to lose 10 lbs. or 100, this is a great starting point. By knowing that you are ready to lose the weight and recognizing that losing the weight will take time and effort, you recognize that you need to make a change. That commitment to making a change is one of the most important steps that you can take to ensuring that you are kept healthy and ready to succeed. All you have to do is commit and then follow through.

From here, it is time to start thinking about the future. If you are serious about this diet, then what you need to do is begin working on yourself. You will need to get through everything that you will need to know and recognize to maintain your own personal health. By looking at how you can change up your own diet and learning how you can make it happen yourself, you should begin to see that losing weight isn't as impossible as you might have thought. Losing weight doesn't need to be difficult or even impossible. It just needs to involve you making a commitment.

Start thinking about your meal plans. What kinds of foods that have been introduced seem enjoyable to you? Which ones are unappealing? Do you have a juicer? These are all considerations that you will need to make to ensure that you are ready to make progress. If you have a list of foods that you are willing to try and that you think will taste good, then you are on the right track! Start putting together your meal plans. Start planning out the right foods that you want to consume and when you will do so. Figure out how to put this all together so that at the end of it all, you will be able to make the changes and commit. When you work hard and plan out how to get the right foods into your diet, you will see the weight start to melt off. You will be able to start making those changes that will be meaningful and provide the success to your weight loss goal.

So, are you ready? Are you going to start taking the leap into the sirtfood diet? Are you ready to commit to losing the weight once and for all? Don't forget what is motivating you to make those changes that you want. Don't forget why you have committed to losing weight. Don't forget to see that you are trying to lose the weight for a reason. When you recognize this, you should be able to maintain the motivation that you will need. From there, all you have to do is get started.

Even if you worry about it, don't forget that you can do this. Don't forget that you are someone who is more than capable of successfully navigating through your diet. Don't forget that you are strong and that you can maintain the motivation that you will need t keep yourself on track. You can do it if you put your mind to it!

Thank you for taking the time to get through this book. Hopefully, as you read, you found that the information that you were given was beneficial to you. Hopefully, you feel ready to tackle your weight loss journey head-on with the sirtfood diet, and hopefully, you feel comfortable with that decision! Finally, if you found that this book was inspiring or beneficial to you, please consider leaving a review on Amazon with your thoughts! Your review and feedback is always greatly appreciated and will help to make sure that future books are even better!